LOW RESIDUE DIET COOKBOOK

A total of 130+ Low-Fiber, Dairy-Free, Nightshade-Free, Specially Designed Stove Top, Oven and Slow Cooker Recipes for Diverticulitis, Ulcerative Colitis, Crohn's Disease & IBD

2 Manuscripts:
Ulcerative Colitis Cookbook
Ulcerative Colitis Cookbook – Slow Cooker

SALLY LLOYD

Copyright © 2018 by SALLY LLOYD.
All rights reserved. This book or any portion thereof may not be reproduced or used in any manner whatsoever without the express written permission of the publisher except for the use of brief quotations in a book review.

This book is not intended as a substitute for the medical advice of physicians. The reader should regularly consult a physician in matters relating to his/her health and particularly with respect to any symptoms that may require diagnosis or medical attention.

No warranties are given in relation to the medical information presented in this Book. No liability will accrue to the writer and/or Book publisher in the event that the reader and/or user suffers any loss as a result of reliance, in part or in full, upon the information presented in this Book.

CONTENT

BREAKFAST & BRUNCH

Sardine-Stuffed Avocado	1
Banana Almond Smoothie	2
Quick Breakfast Pudding	3
Banana Coconut "Oats"	4
Cinnamon Applesauce Oat	5
Pumpkin Porridge	6
Savory Chicken Pancake	7
Turkey Breakfast Sausage	8
Golden Rice Pancake	9
Pumpkin Muffin	10
Almond Pancakes	11
Light Turkey and Oats Casserole	12
Banana Soufflés	13
Apple and Bacon Hash Skillet	14
Mini Spinach Quiche Cup	15
Pumpkin Clafoutis	16
Butternut Squash and Spinach Casserole	17
Smoked Salmon Casserole	18
Coconut Egg Pudding	19
Simple Coconut Bread	20
Cinnamon Banana Squash Bowl	21

SOUPS & STEWS

Thai Chicken Soup	22
Simple Egg Drop Soup	23
Herb Chicken Zoodle Soup	24
Easy Cod Chowder	25
Thai-Style Pumpkin Soup	26
Cream of Mushroom Soup	27
Chicken Avocado Soup	28
Carrot Halibut Soup	29
Creamy Halibut Squash Stew	30
Classic Fish Stock	31
Apple-Butternut Squash Soup	32
Cream of Avocado Salmon Soup	33
Chinese Chicken Rice Porridge	34
Cantonese Fish Congee	35
Turmeric and Ginger Chicken Broth	36
Lemon and Dill Chicken Soup	37

VEGETABLES

Stir Fry Parsnip	38
Cilantro Mashed Carrot	39
Carrot Risotto	40

Braised Kabocha Squash	41
Tender Beet Salad	42
Herb Roasted Beet	43
Sweet and Sour Rutabaga	44
Kale and Squash Gratin	45
Winter Vegetables Casserole	46

POULTRY RECIPES

Chinese Fried Rice	47
Avocado Chicken Zoodle	48
Chicken Piccata	49
Creamy Cilantro and Lime Chicken	50
Indonesian Peanut Coconut Chicken	51
Herb Roasted Chicken	52
Spaghetti Squash Turkey Alfredo	53
Hariyali Chicken Tikka	54
Simple Teriyaki Chicken	55
Apple Lemon Chicken	56
Chicken Biryani	57
Chicken Schawarma	58

FISH RECIPES

Simple Salmon Cake	59
Mackerel with Herb Sauce	60
Salmon in Creamed Spinach	61
Creamy Turmeric Cod	62
Lime and Ginger Salmon	63
Herbes de Provence Salmon Zoodle	64
Baked Cod with Zucchini	65
Sweet and Sour Glazed Salmon	66
French Salt Cod Brandade	67
Citrus and Sage Salmon	68
Gefilte Fish	69

DESSERT & SNACK

Roasted Butternut Squash Hummus	70
Almond Butter Ice Cream	71
Wild salmon Paté	72
Cinnamon Coconut Pudding	73
Spaghetti Squash Hash Browns	74
Mini Pumpkin Banana Pie	75
Coconut Rice Pudding	76
Rice Crackers with Herbs	77
Apple Coconut Butter Cup	78
Banana Coconut Ice Cream	79
Carrot Coconut Truffles	80
Coconut Plantain Macaron	81

SLOW COOKER

BREAKFAST

Oat-Stuffed Apples	83
Pumpkin Pie Oatmeal	84
Chinese Chicken Congee	85
Butternut Squash apple Oatmeal	86
Turkey Breakfast Casserole	87
Peanut Butter Breakfast Bar	88

SOUPS & BROTHS

Greek Chicken Soup	89
Classic Chicken and Rice Soup	90
Lemony Kale Chicken Soup	91
Curry Pumpkin Carrot Soup	92
Turmeric Bone Broth	93

SIDE DISH

Thyme Butter Rice	94
Butternut Squash Risotto	95
Rosemary Acorn Squash	96

DESSERT

Simple Plantain Mash	97
Coconut Rice Pudding	98
Pumpkin Butter	99
Blackberry Jam	100
Cranberry Orange Sauce	101
Pear Butter	102
Classic Apple Sauce	103
Coconut Yogurt	104

CHICKEN

Lemon Cilantro Chicken and Rice	105
Chicken Rice Casserole	106
Chicken Stroganoff	107
Moroccan Chicken Drumsticks	108
Pear Cranberry Squash Chicken	109
Mild Chicken Carnitas	110
Balsamic Chicken Thighs	111
Apple Acorn Squash Chicken	112
Lemon Rosemary Chicken	113
Thai Roast Chicken	114
Teriyaki Chicken	115
Fennel Orange Chicken	116
Thai Peanut Chicken	117
Bourbon Chicken	118
Chicken Tikka Masala	119
Hawaiian Pineapple Chicken	120

BEEF, LAMB AND PORK

Only for those who can tolerate

Mongolian beef	121
Beef Bourguignon	122
Classic Pot Roast	123
Italian Roasted Beef	124
Minty Lamb Shanks	125
Simple Lamb Curry	126
Apple Squash Lamb Stew	127
Lemon Rosemary Lamb	128
Honey Ginger Lime Pork	129
Maple Balsamic Pork	130
Apple Rosemary Pork Roast	131
Cuban Pork	132

BREAKFAST & BRUNCH
SARDINE-STUFFED AVOCADO

INGREDENTS

1 large avocado, seed removed and cut in half

1 3.75-ounce can sardines in water, drained

1 tablespoon mayonnaise

1 tablespoon fresh lemon juice

1/4 teaspoon turmeric

1/4 teaspoon salt

PREP TIME
5 MINUTES

COOK TIME
NA

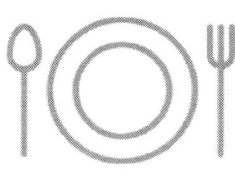

SERVES
2

DIRECTIONS

1. Scoop out the avocado flesh, leaving a 1/2 inch on the inside.

2. Put the avocado flesh, sardines, mayonnaise and turmeric in a small bowl. Use a fork to mash until well incorporated.

3. Season with lemon juice and sea salt. Add the mixture back to the avocado and serve.

BREAKFAST & BRUNCH
BANANA ALMOND SMOOTHIE

PREP TIME
5 MINUTES

COOK TIME
NA

SERVES
2

INGREDENTS

2 cups unsweetened coconut milk

1 medium frozen banana

3 tablespoons smooth almond butter

DIRECTIONS

1. Blend all ingredients and serve.

BREAKFAST & BRUNCH
QUICK BREAKFAST PUDDING

INGREDIENTS

1/2 cup pumpkin puree

1/2 cup pureed pears or applesauce

1 tablespoon of nut butter of choice

Honey or stevia to taste

PREP TIME
5 MINUTES

COOK TIME
NA

DIRECTIONS

1. Mix well and add honey/stevia to taste.

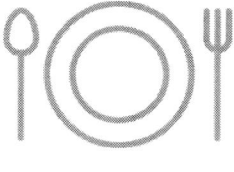

SERVES
1

BREAKFAST & BRUNCH
BANANA COCONUT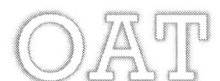

INGREDIENTS

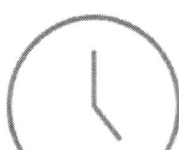

PREP TIME
5 MINUTES

COOK TIME
10 MINUTES

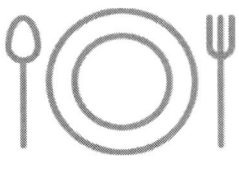

SERVES
2

1 medium ripe banana, peeled and sliced

1/2 cup unsweetened coconut flakes or shredded coconut

1/3 cup coconut milk or almond milk

1/3 cup coconut cream

2 tablespoons nut butter of choice

1 tablespoon maple syrup (substitute with stevia if can't tolerate)

1 teaspoon cinnamon

1/4 teaspoon vanilla extract

Fat-free cooking spray

DIRECTIONS

1. In a medium bowl, combine all ingredients except banana.
2. In a pan, cook the banana until soft. Mash the banana.
3. Stir in the mixture until hot.

BREAKFAST & BRUNCH
CINNAMON APPLESAUCE OAT

INGREDENTS

1 cup instant oats

2 cups water

3/4 cup applesauce

3/4 teaspoon cinnamon

1/2 teaspoon turmeric

1/2 teaspoon vanilla extract

Maple syrup to taste

PREP TIME
NA

COOK TIME
15 MINUTES

DIRECTIONS

1. In a sauce pan, add oats, water, cinnamon, turmeric and vanilla extract. Bring it to a boil and then reduce to low heat.

2. Simmer until the oats are soft. Add applesauce and sweeten with maple syrup to taste.

3. Serve immediately.

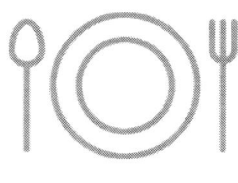

SERVES
4

BREAKFAST & BRUNCH
PUMPKIN PORRIDGE

PREP TIME
5 MINUTES

COOK TIME
10 MINUTES

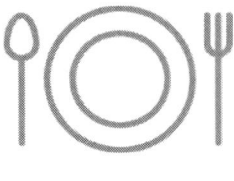

SERVES
6

INGREDIENTS

1 15-ounce can pumpkin puree

3 cups coconut milk

1/3 cup coconut flour

2 tablespoons gelatin

2 tablespoons maple syrup

1 teaspoon vanilla extract

Pinch of salt

DIRECTIONS

1. In a sauce pan, add a cup of coconut milk and the gelatin. Let it sit for 5 minutes.

2. In a mixing bowl, combine pumpkin puree, the rest of the coconut milk, coconut flour and salt.

3. Heat the gelatin mixture on low heat until it melts. Add the maple syrup and stir well.

4. Add the gelatin mixture to the pumpkin mixture. Add vanilla extract.

5. Stir until well combined and serve.

BREAKFAST & BRUNCH
SAVORY CHICKEN PANCAKE

INGREDENTS

2 ounces leftover chicken

2 large eggs

1/3 cup pumpkin puree

1 tablespoon coconut oil

1 teaspoon chopped fresh parsley

Pinch of salt

PREP TIME
5 MINUTES

COOK TIME
10 MINUTES

DIRECTIONS

1. Using a food processor, combine chicken, pumpkin puree, parsley and eggs.

2. In a skillet, add oil and heat until melted. Scoop the mixture and spread to form pancakes. Cook until golden brown on both sides, flipping halfway through.

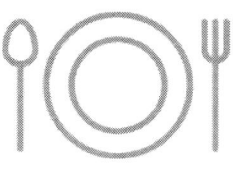

SERVES
2

BREAKFAST & BRUNCH
TURKEY BREAKFAST SAUSAGE

PREP TIME
10 MINUTES

COOK TIME
10 MINUTES

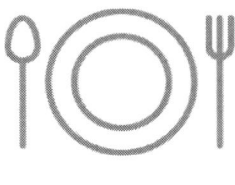

SERVES
4

INGREDIENTS

- 1 pound lean ground turkey
- 1 teaspoon sage, rubbed
- 1/2 teaspoon salt
- 1/2 teaspoon dried thyme
- 1/8 teaspoon ground cloves
- 1/8 teaspoon nutmeg
- Fat-free cooking spray

DIRECTIONS

1. In a mixing bowl, combine all ingredients. Divide the mixture and shape into 8 patties.

2. In a pan, cook the patties over medium heat for 5 minutes per side or until cooked through.

BREAKFAST & BRUNCH
GOLDEN RICE PANCAKE

INGREDIENTS

1 cup cooked white rice

1 large egg, beaten

1/4 cup sliced scallion (omit if can't tolerate)

1/4 teaspoon turmeric

1/4 teaspoon ground ginger

1/4 teaspoon salt

Fat-free cooking spray

PREP TIME
5 MINUTES

COOK TIME
15 MINUTES

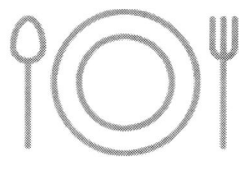

SERVES
5

DIRECTIONS

1. In a mixing bowl, stir all ingredients together.
2. Cook the pancakes in a skillet until golden brown, about 3-4 minutes each side.

BREAKFAST & BRUNCH
PUMPKIN MUFFIN

INGREDIENTS

PREP TIME
5 MINUTES

- 3/4 cup coconut flour
- 1/2 cup pumpkin puree
- 1/2 cup maple syrup (substitute with stevia if can't tolerate)
- 6 large eggs
- 1 teaspoon fresh lemon juice
- 3/4 teaspoon baking soda
- 1/2 teaspoon ground ginger
- 1/4 teaspoon ground cloves

COOK TIME
30 MINUTES

DIRECTIONS

1. Preheat the oven to 350 °F.
2. In a mixing bowl, slightly beat the eggs and then stir in all the ingredients. Mix until well incorporated.
3. Divide the mixture into 12 baking cups. Bake for 25-30 minutes.

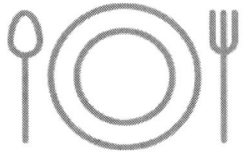

SERVES
12

BREAKFAST & BRUNCH
ALMOND PANCAKE

INGREDIENTS

- 1 cup almond flour
- 1/2 cup applesauce
- 4 large eggs, separated
- 1 teaspoon cinnamon
- 1/2 teaspoon nutmeg
- Fat-free cooking spray

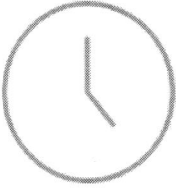

PREP TIME
5 MINUTES

COOK TIME
20 MINUTES

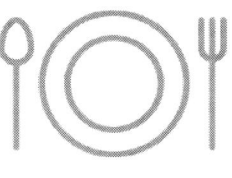

SERVES
3

DIRECTIONS

1. In a mixing bowl, mix the almond flour, yolks, applesauce and spices.
2. In another bowl, beat the egg white until stiff. Then gently fold in the batter.
3. Cook the pancakes in batches.

BREAKFAST & BRUNCH
LIGHT TURKEY AND OATS CASSEROLE

PREP TIME
5 MINUTES

COOK TIME
25 MINUTES

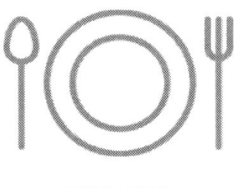

SERVES
4

INGREDIENTS

8 slices extra-lean turkey Bacon, chopped

2 cups liquid egg whites

1/2 cup instant oats

1/4 teaspoon salt

Fat-free cooking spray

DIRECTIONS

1. Preheat the oven to 350 °F. Spray an 8"x8" square pan.

2. In a large bowl, mix together 3/4 of bacon and all other ingredients together. Pour half of the mixture into the baking pan. Bake for 20 minutes.

3. Add the remaining mixture and top with the remaining bacon. Bake for 20-25 minutes or until the center is set.

BREAKFAST & BRUNCH
BANANA SOUFFLÉS

INGREDIENTS

2 medium ripe bananas, peeled

6 large eggs, yolks and whites separated

2 tablespoons maple syrup (substitute with stevia if can't tolerate)

1/2 teaspoon vanilla extract

Fat-free cooking spray

PREP TIME
15 MINUTES

COOK TIME
15 MINUTES

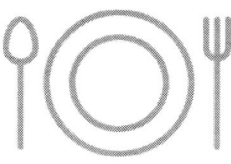

SERVES
6

DIRECTIONS

1. Preheat the oven to 400 °F.
2. In a small bowl, mash the bananas and stir in the syrup.
3. Beat the egg whites to soft peaks. Then slowly add the yolks and banana mixture while folding gently.
4. Divide the mixture into 6 greased ramekins.
5. Bake for 15 minutes.

BREAKFAST & BRUNCH
APPLE AND BACON HASH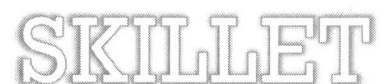

INGREDENTS

6 ounces extra lean turkey Bacon, diced

1 large sweet potato, peeled and cut into 1/2-inch cubes

1 large apple, peeled, seeded and cut into 1/2-inch cubes

2 tablespoons chopped fresh parsley

1 tablespoon coconut oil

1 tablespoon minced fresh sage

1 teaspoon cinnamon

Salt to taste

PREP TIME
10 MINUTES

COOK TIME
25 MINUTES

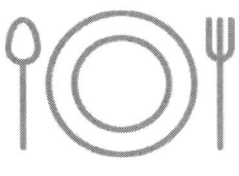

SERVES
3

DIRECTIONS

1. In a skillet, add the oil and cook the bacon over medium heat for about 3 minutes. Set the bacon aside. Leave the fat in the skillet.

2. Add apple and cinnamon. Cook for about 7 minutes or until soft. Set aside.

3. Add sweet potato and 1 tablespoon of water. Cover the lid immediately and cook for 2 minutes. Stir and repeat the previous step and allow to cook for another 2 minutes. Keep cooking while stirring until soft.

4. Add the apple, bacon and the herbs. Season with salt and cook until warm throughout.

BREAKFAST & BRUNCH
MINI SPINACH QUICHE

INGREDENTS

- 10 ounces fresh baby spinach
- 4 large eggs
- 8 ounces baby portabella mushrooms, roughly chopped (omit if can't tolerate)
- 2 tablespoons coconut cream
- 1 tablespoon minced fresh basil
- 1 tablespoon minced fresh parsley
- 1/2 teaspoon salt
- Fat-free cooking spray

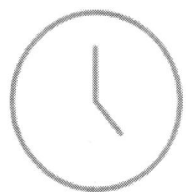

PREP TIME
5 MINUTES

COOK TIME
45 MINUTES

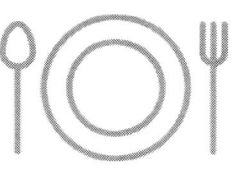

SERVES
12

DIRECTIONS

1. Preheat the oven to 350 °F.
2. In a pan, sauté the mushrooms over medium heat for 5-6 minutes until lightly browned. Set aside.
3. Sauté the spinach for 3-4 minutes until wilted. Drain the excess water.
4. In a mixing bowl, slightly beat the eggs then add cooked vegetables and the rest of the ingredients. Mix well.
5. Divide the mixture into 12 baking cups. Bake for 20-25 minutes or until the centers are set.

BREAKFAST & BRUNCH
PUMPKIN CLAFOUTIS

PREP TIME
5 MINUTES

COOK TIME
45 MINUTES

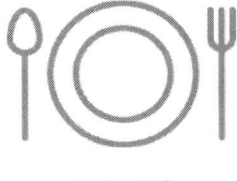

SERVES
6

INGREDIENTS

4 large eggs

1 3/4 cups pumpkin puree

1/2 cup coconut oil, melted

1/2 cup coconut milk

1/3 cup maple syrup or to taste (substitute with stevia if can't tolerate)

1/3 cup almond flour

2 teaspoons vanilla extract

1 teaspoon cinnamon

1/2 teaspoon ground ginger

1/4 teaspoon salt

Pinch of nutmeg

Fat-free cooking spray

DIRECTIONS

1. Preheat the oven to 325 °F.

2. Blend all ingredients using a food processor or blender.

3. Spray an 8"x8" baking dish. Pour the mixture in and bake for 35-45 minutes or until center is set.

BREAKFAST & BRUNCH
BUTTERNUT SQUASH AND SPINACH CASSEROLE

INGREDIENTS

1 3/4 cups liquid egg whites

2 cups chopped spinach

1 cup chopped butternut squash, finely cubed

1 teaspoon dried basil

1/4 teaspoon salt

Fat-free cooking spray

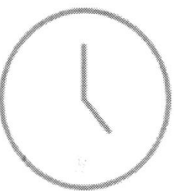

PREP TIME
10 MINUTES

COOK TIME
50 MINUTES

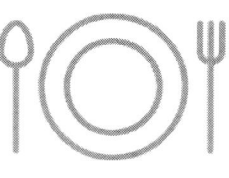

SERVES
8

DIRECTIONS

1. Preheat the oven to 350 °F. Spray a 9" round pan.

2. Spray ovenproof pan and sauté butternut squash over medium heat until slightly brown, about 5 minutes. Then add in Spinach and sauté until completely wilted. Pour into the baking pan.

3. In a measuring cup, mix egg white and seasoning together then pour into the baking pan.

4. Bake for 35-40 minutes or until center is set.

BREAKFAST & BRUNCH
SMOKED SALMON 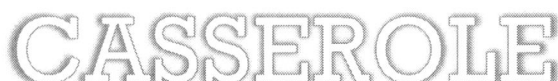 CASSEROLE

INGREDIENTS

PREP TIME
20 MINUTES

3 medium zucchini, shredded

8 large eggs

4 ounces smoked salmon

1 teaspoon dried dill

1 teaspoon salt

Fat-free cooking spray

COOK TIME
40 MINUTES

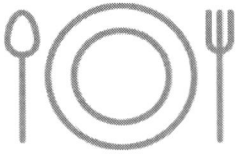

SERVES
6

DIRECTIONS

1. Preheat the oven to 350 °F.

2. In a pan, sauté the zucchini over medium heat for 6-8 minutes until lightly browned. Season with salt. Drain the excess water and set aside to cool.

3. In a large bowl, beat the egg slightly and add dill and smoked salmon. Add the cooled zucchini and mix well.

4. Pour the mixture into an 8"x8" greased baking dish. Bake for 30-35 minutes or until the center is set.

BREAKFAST & BRUNCH
COCONUT EGG PUDDING

INGREDIENTS

6 large eggs

3 cups coconut milk

1/2 cup maple syrup

(substitute with stevia if can't tolerate)

1 teaspoon vanilla extract

1/4 teaspoon salt

Pinch of nutmeg

Fat-free cooking spray

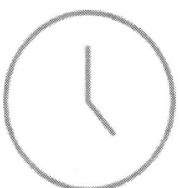

PREP TIME
10 MINUTES

COOK TIME
50 MINUTES

DIRECTIONS

1. Preheat the oven to 400 °F.
2. In a mixing bowl, slightly beat the eggs until combined.
3. Add the rest of the ingredients and mix well.
4. Divide the mixture into 12 baking cups. Bake for 45-50 minutes or until the centers are set.

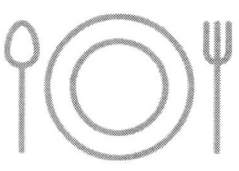

SERVES
12

BREAKFAST & BRUNCH
SIMPLE COCONUT BREAD

PREP TIME
15 MINUTES

COOK TIME
50 MINUTES

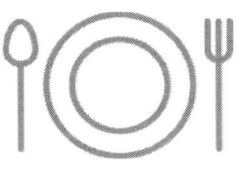

SERVES
12

INGREDENTS

1 1/8 cups coconut butter, melted

1/4 cup coconut oil, melted

5 large eggs, yolks and whites separated

1/2 teaspoon salt

3/4 teaspoon baking soda

Fat-free cooking spray

DIRECTIONS

1. Preheat the oven to 300 °F.
2. Beat the egg whites to soft peaks.
3. Add the egg yolks one by one and then the rest of the ingredients. Mix until well incorporated.
4. Spray a 9"x5" loaf pan. Pour the mixture into the pan. Bake for 40-50 minutes or until the center is set.

BREAKFAST & BRUNCH
CINNAMON BANANA SQUASH BOWL

INGREDENTS

1/2 large spaghetti squash, seeds removed

1 1/4 cups shredded coconut

2 1/2 cups coconut milk

1 large ripe banana, peeled and mashed

1 teaspoon cinnamon

Salt to taste

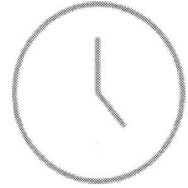

PREP TIME
60 MINUTES

COOK TIME
10 MINUTES

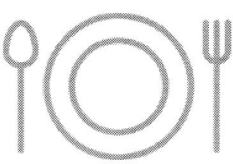

SERVES
4

DIRECTIONS

1. On the night before, bake the spaghetti squash in 1/2 inch of water for 50-60 minutes at 350 °F. Let it cool and then refrigerate overnight.

2. The next morning, cut the spaghetti squash into chunks. Add all ingredients in a sauce pan. Cook in medium heat until boiling then reduce to low heat and simmer for 5 minutes.

3. Blend the mixture into desired consistency and serve.

SOUPS & STEWS
THAI CHICKEN SOUP

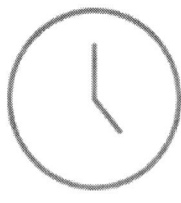

PREP TIME
5 MINUTES

COOK TIME
10 MINUTES

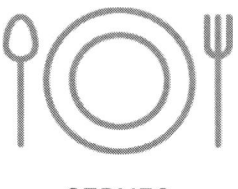

SERVES
3

INGREDIENTS

6 ounces leftover chicken, shredded

3 cups chicken broth, preferably homemade

1 cup coconut milk

1 cup sliced mushrooms (optional)

1 medium carrot, peeled and julienned

2 tablespoons fresh lime juice

1 teaspoon ground ginger

Salt to taste

DIRECTIONS

1. In a pot, bring the broth and ginger to a boil then reduce to low. Simmer for 5 minutes.

2. Add chicken, coconut milk, mushrooms and carrots. Season with salt. Cook until the carrots and mushrooms are soft.

3. Add lime juice before serving.

SOUPS & STEWS
SIMPLE EGG DROP SOUP

INGREDENTS

4 cups chicken broth, preferably homemade

2 cups fresh baby spinach

2 large eggs, beaten

4 tablespoons soy sauce or coconut amino

1 tablespoon sesame oil

Salt to taste

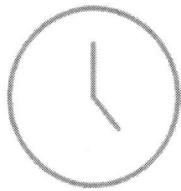

PREP TIME
5 MINUTES

COOK TIME
10 MINUTES

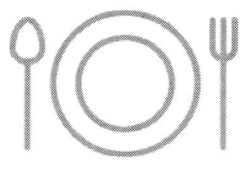

SERVES
2

DIRECTIONS

1. In a pot, add broth, spinach, soy sauce and oil. Bring to a boil. Season with salt.

2. Slowly add the eggs while stirring constantly. Remove from heat and serve immediately.

SOUPS & STEWS
HERB CHICKEN ZOODLE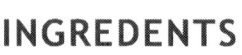

PREP TIME
10 MINUTES

COOK TIME
10 MINUTES

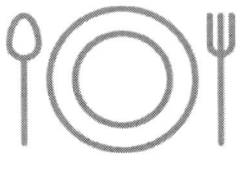

SERVES
4

INGREDIENTS

8 ounces leftover chicken, shredded

4 cups chicken broth, preferably homemade

2 medium zucchini, spiralized

1 medium carrot, peeled and julienned

1/2 teaspoon finely chopped rosemary

1/2 teaspoon finely chopped thyme

1/2 teaspoon finely chopped parsley

Salt to taste

Fat-free cooking spray

DIRECTIONS

1. In a large pot, sauté the carrot until soft.
2. Add broth and herbs. Bring to a boil. Season with salt.
3. Add Zoodle and chicken. Heat until cooked through.

SOUPS & STEWS
EASY COD CHOWDER

INGREDENTS

12 ounces wild cod, cut into pieces

8 ounces extra-lean turkey Bacon, cooked and diced

3 cups chicken broth, preferably homemade

1 13.5-ounce can coconut milk

2 medium carrots, peeled and julienned

1 large leek, chopped (optional)

1 1/2 tablespoons coconut flour

1 bay leaf

1 teaspoon turmeric

1/2 teaspoon coriander

1/2 teaspoon salt

Fat-free cooking spray

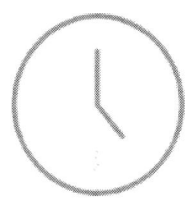

PREP TIME
10 MINUTES

COOK TIME
20 MINUTES

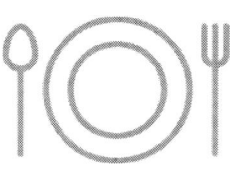

SERVES
6

DIRECTIONS

1. In a large pot, sauté the leek and carrot until soft. Then sprinkle coconut flour and heat for 30 seconds while stirring.

2. Add the rest of the ingredients. Bring to a boil and then reduce to low heat. Simmer for about 10 minutes or until cod is cooked through.

3. Top with turkey bacon and serve.

SOUPS & STEWS
THAI-STYLE PUMPKIN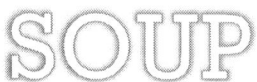

PREP TIME
10 MINUTES

COOK TIME
20 MINUTES

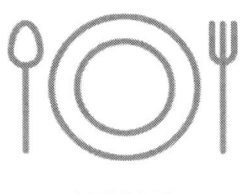

SERVES
6

INGREDENTS

2 cups pumpkin puree

5 cups chicken broth, preferably homemade

1 cup coconut milk

1 tablespoon fish sauce

1 tablespoon lime juice

1 teaspoon ginger

1 teaspoon honey

1/2 teaspoon salt

DIRECTIONS

1. In a large pot, add broth, pumpkin puree, fish sauce and salt. Bring to to a boil and then reduce to low heat. Simmer for 15 minutes.

2. Stir in coconut milk and lime juice. Remove from heat. Blend in small batches and serve.

SOUPS & STEWS
CREAM OF MUSHROOM SOUP

INGREDIENTS

1 1/2 pounds wild mushrooms, sliced

7 cups chicken broth, preferably homemade

1 cup coconut milk

1 tablespoon chopped fresh thyme

Salt to taste

Fat-free cooking spray

PREP TIME
15 MINUTES

COOK TIME
25 MINUTES

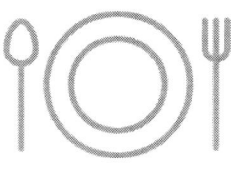

SERVES
4

DIRECTIONS

1. In a large pot, sauté the mushrooms and thyme until fragrant.
2. Add broth. Bring to a boil and then reduce to low heat. Simmer for 25 minutes.
3. Add coconut milk. Season with salt.
4. Blend the soup in batches and serve.

SOUPS & STEWS
CHICKEN AVOCADO SOUP

PREP TIME
10 MINUTES

COOK TIME
30 MINUTES

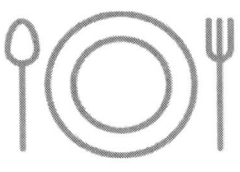

SERVES
4

INGREDENTS

- 2 skinless chicken breasts
- 2 avocados, seeds and skin removed, diced
- 6 cups chicken broth, preferably homemade
- 1 cup chopped green onion (Optional)
- 1/2 cup finely chopped cilantro
- 1/8 teaspoon cumin
- Salt to taste
- Fat-free cooking spray

DIRECTIONS

1. In a sauce pan, grill the chicken until cooked through. Remove from heat and shred into small pieces.
2. In a large pot, sauté the green onion until soft. Add broth, cumin and salt. Bring to a boil then reduce to low heat.
3. Heat for another 15 minutes.
4. Meanwhile, divide the shredded chicken, avocados and chopped cilantro into 4 bowls. Pour the hot soup and serve.

SOUPS & STEWS
CARROT HALIBUT SOUP

INGREDENTS

1 pound halibut, cut into 1-inch pieces

6 medium carrots, peeled and sliced

2 cups chicken broth, preferably homemade

1 cup water

1 tablespoon minced fresh ginger

Salt to taste

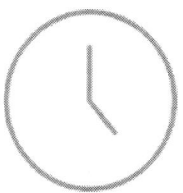

PREP TIME
10 MINUTES

COOK TIME
30 MINUTES

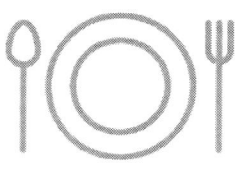

SERVES
6

DIRECTIONS

1. In a large pot, add carrots, ginger, broth and water. Bring to a boil and then reduce to low heat. Simmer for 20 minutes.

2. Blend the soup. Return to the pot. Add halibut. Cook until halibut is cooked through. Season with salt and serve.

SOUPS & STEWS
CREAMY HALIBUT SQUASH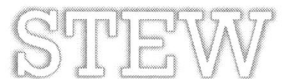

PREP TIME
15 MINUTES

COOK TIME
45 MINUTES

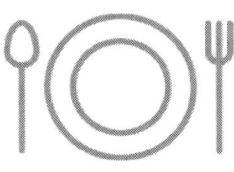

SERVES
6

INGREDENTS

1 pound skinless chicken breasts, cut into 1-inch pieces

1 large leek, white parts only, sliced

3 medium carrots, peeled and diced

1 medium celeriac, peeled and sliced

1 tablespoon chopped fresh thyme

1 cup chicken broth, preferably homemade

1/3 cup coconut milk

1 teaspoon salt

Fat-free cooking spray

DIRECTIONS

1. In a large pot, brown the chicken over medium heat and season with salt, about 5 minutes.

2. Add all the vegetables. Stir and cook the vegetables until fragrant.

3. Add stock and thyme. Bring to boil and reduce to low heat. Simmer for 30 minutes, half-covered.

4. Stir in coconut milk and stir well. Remove from heat and serve.

SOUPS & STEWS
CLASSIC FISH STOCK

INGREDENTS

1 pound fish bones from bass, flounder or halibut, cut into pieces and clean off all the blood

2 medium carrots, peeled and chopped

7 cups water

1 bay leaf

2 tablespoons chopped fresh parsley

2 tablespoons chopped fresh thyme

1 teaspoon salt

PREP TIME
10 MINUTES

COOK TIME
50 MINUTES

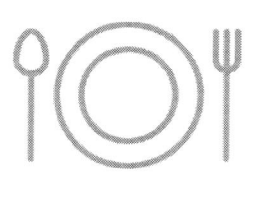

SERVES
6

DIRECTIONS

1. Add water to a large pot. Bring it a boil. Add ginger root and fish bones. Boil over high heat for 10 minutes.

2. Add carrot. Once boiled, reduce to low heat. Cover and simmer for 40 minutes. Add salt and herbs.

SOUPS & STEWS
APPLE-BUTTERNUT SQUASH SOUP

PREP TIME
10 MINUTES

COOK TIME
50 MINUTES

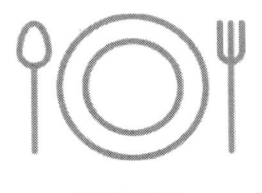

SERVES
4

INGREDIENTS

1 medium butternut squash, peeled, seeded and diced

1 medium apple, peeled, cored and sliced

4 cups chicken broth, preferably homemade

1 teaspoon cinnamon

1/2 teaspoon salt

Fat-free cooking spray

DIRECTIONS

1. In a large pot, sauté squash, apple and seasoning for 10 minutes.

2. Add broth. Bring to a boil then reduce to low heat. Simmer for 30 minutes.

3. Blend the soup in small batches and serve.

SOUPS & STEWS
CREAM OF AVOCADO SALMON SOUP

INGREDENTS

3 avocados, seeds and skin removed

1 6-ounce can wild caught salmon, rinsed and drained

1 1/2 cups chicken broth, preferably homemade

2 tablespoons coconut cream

1 tablespoon fresh lemon juice

Salt to taste

PREP TIME
65 MINUTES

COOK TIME
NA

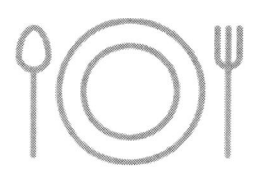

SERVES
3

DIRECTIONS

1. Blend avocado, broth, coconut cream, lemon juice and salt using a blender until smooth.
2. Refrigerate for 1 hour.
3. Divide the soup into 3 servings. Top with salmon and serve.

SOUPS & STEWS
CHINESE CHICKEN RICE PORRIDGE

PREP TIME
10 MINUTES

COOK TIME
60 MINUTES

SERVES
4

INGREDIENTS

3/4 cup uncooked white rice, rinsed and drained

10 cups chicken broth, preferably homemade

2 skinless chicken breasts, cut into thin stripes

Soy sauce/coconut amino and sesame oil, for serving (optional)

Salt to taste

DIRECTIONS

1. In a large pot, add the rice. chicken and broth. Bring to a boil and then reduce to low heat.

2. Simmer for 1 hour half-covered, while scraping the bottom and stirring every 20 minutes.

3. Season with salt before serving.

SOUPS & STEWS
CANTONESE FISH CONGEE

INGREDIENTS

1 pound white fish, thinly sliced

10 cups water

1 1/2 cups uncooked white rice, rinsed and drained

1 tablespoon soy sauce or coconut amino

1 teaspoon sesame oil

1 teaspoon ground ginger

Salt to taste

PREP TIME
10 MINUTES

COOK TIME
60 MINUTES

SERVES
6

DIRECTIONS

1. In a bowl, mix fish, soy sauce, ginger and sesame oil. Set aside to marinate for 30 minutes.

2. In a large pot, add water and rice. Bring to a boil and then reduce to low heat.

3. Simmer for 30 minutes half-covered, while scraping the bottom and stirring every 15 minutes.

4. Add the fish and bring the congee to a boil. Heat for 3-5 more minutes until fish is cooked through. Season with salt and serve.

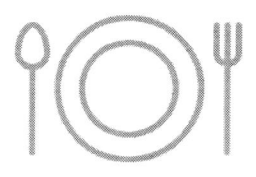

SOUPS & STEWS
TURMERIC AND GINGER CHICKEN BROTH

INGREDIENTS

1 pound bone-in chicken pieces

10 shallots, peeled

2 medium carrots, peeled and chopped

8 cups water

2 tablespoons grated fresh ginger root

1 tablespoon ground turmeric

1/2 teaspoon salt

PREP TIME
15 MINUTES

COOK TIME
75 MINUTES

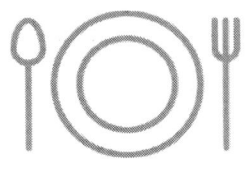

SERVES
6

DIRECTIONS

1. In a large pot, add 3-4 cups of water. Bring it to a boil. Blanch the chicken for 5 minutes.

2. Discard the water. Rinse the chicken to remove surface impurities.

3. Add water, chicken, spices and all vegetables to the pot. Bring it to a boil. Then reduce to low heat. Cover and simmer for 65 minutes. Skim off the fat on the surface. Add salt.

SOUPS & STEWS
LEMON AND DILL CHICKEN SOUP

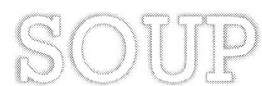

INGREDIENTS

1 pound bone-in chicken pieces

3 medium carrots, diced

1 lemon, juice only

10 cups water

1 bay leaf

2 tablespoons chopped fresh dill

1/2 teaspoon salt

PREP TIME
15 MINUTES

COOK TIME
75 MINUTES

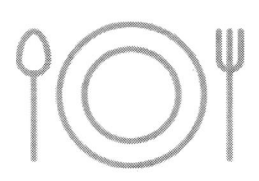

SERVES
6

DIRECTIONS

1. In a large pot, add 3-4 cups of water. Bring it to a boil. Blanch the chicken for 5 minutes.

2. Discard the water. Rinse the chicken to remove surface impurities.

3. Add all ingredients except dill and salt. Bring it to a boil. Cover and simmer for 55 minutes.

4. Skim off the fat on the surface. Add dill and salt. Simmer for another 10 minutes.

VEGETABLE STIR FRY PARSNIP

PREP TIME
10 MINUTES

COOK TIME
10 MINUTES

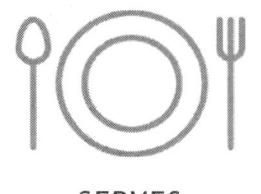

SERVES
3

INGREDIENTS

- 3 large parsnips, peeled and julienned
- 1 tablespoon extra-virgin olive oil
- 1/4 teaspoon ground ginger
- 1/4 teaspoon turmeric
- Pinch of salt
- Soy sauce and sesame oil, for serving (optional)

DIRECTIONS

1. In a sauce pan, add oil and parsnip. Sauté over medium heat until fragrant.
2. Add ginger, turmeric and salt. Stir well and serve immediately.

VEGETABLE
CILANTRO MASHED CARROT

INGREDENTS

6 medium carrots, peeled and roughly chopped

1/2 cup chopped cilantro

1/3 cup coconut milk

2 tablespoons extra virgin olive oil

1 teaspoon salt

PREP TIME
5 MINUTES

COOK TIME
20 MINUTES

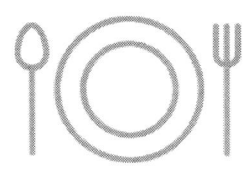

SERVES
4

DIRECTIONS

1. In a large pot, add carrots and add enough water to cover. Bring it to a boil and reduce to low heat. Boil for about 15 minutes or until carrots are tender. Drain throughly.

2. In a food processor, add all ingredients and blend until smooth.

VEGETABLE CARROT RISOTTO

PREP TIME
5 MINUTES

COOK TIME
25 MINUTES

SERVES
4

INGREDIENTS

6 medium carrots, peeled and roughly chopped

1 cup chicken broth, preferably homemade

2 tablespoons extra virgin olive oil

1/4 cup chopped fresh mint

1 tablespoon chopped fresh parsley

1 teaspoon salt

DIRECTIONS

1. Use a food processor to blend the carrot into rice-sized pieces.

2. In a sauce pan, add oil and carrot. Sauté for 5 minutes.

3. Add broth, herbs and salt. Bring to a boil then reduce to low heat. Simmer for 20 minutes or until the carrot is tender.

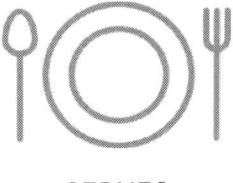

VEGETABLE
BRAISED KABOCHA SQUASH

INGREDIENTS

1/2 medium kabocha squash, peeled, seeded and sliced into 1/4-inch wedges

1/4 cup chicken broth

1/2-inch fresh ginger, minced

3 tablespoons soy sauce or coconut amino

2 tablespoons sesame oil

1 tablespoon maple syrup

PREP TIME
10 MINUTES

COOK TIME
25 MINUTES

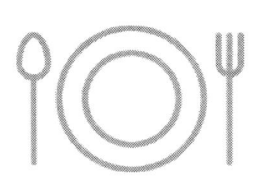

SERVES
6

DIRECTIONS

1. In a pan, add oil and sauté ginger until fragrant. Add broth, soy sauce/coconut amino and syrup. Bring to a simmer.

2. Add squash and cook for 4 minutes on each side. Cover and cook for another 15 minutes, turning occasionally.

3. Serve with white rice if desired.

VEGETABLE
TENDER BEET SALAD

INGREDIENTS

6 medium beets (skin on), washed

1/4 cup chopped fresh dill

3 tablespoons extra virgin olive oil

1 tablespoon apple cider vinegar

1 teaspoon fish sauce

1/2 teaspoon salt

PREP TIME
10 MINUTES

COOK TIME
45 MINUTES

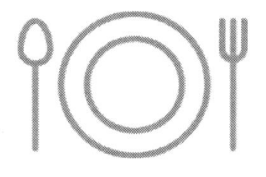

SERVES
4

DIRECTIONS

1. In a large pot, add beets and enough water to cover. Bring it to a boil and reduce to low heat. Boil for about 30 minutes or until beets are tender. Set aside to cool.

2. In a small bowl, combine oil, vinegar, fish sauce and salt.

3. Peel and chop the beets into bite-sized pieces.

4. In a mixing bowl, toss dressing, beets and fresh dill together and serve.

VEGETABLE
HERB ROASTED BEET

INGREDIENTS

6 medium beets (skin on), washed and chopped

1 tablespoon extra virgin olive oil

1/2 teaspoon Herbes de Provence

1/4 teaspoon salt

PREP TIME
10 MINUTES

COOK TIME
50 MINUTES

SERVES
4

DIRECTIONS

1. Preheat the oven to 350 °F.

2. In a mixing bowl, mix all ingredients. Spread the beets on a baking dish. Bake for 45 minutes or until tender.

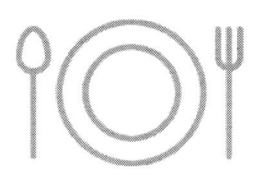

VEGETABLE
SWEET AND SOUR RUTABAGA

PREP TIME
10 MINUTES

COOK TIME
50 MINUTES

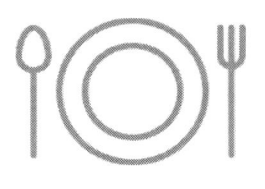

SERVES
4

INGREDENTS

1/2 large rutabaga, cut into 1-inch cubes

2 tablespoons extra virgin olive oil, divided

1 tablespoon maple syrup

1 tablespoon lemon juice

1 tablespoon chopped fresh thyme

1/2 teaspoon salt

DIRECTIONS

1. Preheat the oven to 400 °F.

2. Line a baking dish with parchment paper. Toss rutabaga, 1 tablespoon of oil and salt together and spread evenly. Roast the rutabaga for 40 minutes, turning halfway through.

3. In a small bowl, combine remaining oil, syrup, lemon juice and thyme.

4. Take out the baking dish and drizzle the glaze on top. Bake for another 10 minutes.

VEGETABLE
KALE AND SQUASH GRATIN

INGREDENTS

2 1/2 pounds butternut squash, peeled, seeded and sliced into 1/8-inch wedges

1 13.5-ounce can coconut milk

A bunch of kale, stemmed and roughly-chopped

5 tablespoons extra virgin olive oil

2 teaspoons of ground cinnamon

Pinch of nutmeg

1 teaspoon salt

PREP TIME
15 MINUTES

COOK TIME
45 MINUTES

SERVES
8

DIRECTIONS

1. Preheat the oven to 400 °F.
2. Spread 1 tablespoon of oil on an 8"x8" baking dish.
3. In a pot, add all ingredients. Cook over medium heat for 10-15 minutes until the squash is a little tender.
4. Transfer to the baking dish and spread evenly. Bake for 20-30 minutes or until golden brown on top and cooked through.

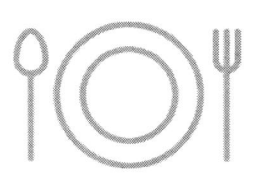

VEGETABLE
WINTER VEGETABLES AND HERBS CASSEROLE

INGREDENTS

- 3 medium zucchini, peeled and diced
- 3 cups diced winter squash
- 3 cups peeled and diced carrots
- 2 cups peeled and diced parsnip
- 2 cups peeled and diced rutabaga
- 2 cups chicken broth
- 1 cup white wine (replace with broth if can't tolerate)
- 2 tablespoons extra virgin olive oil
- 1 tablespoon finely chopped fresh parsley
- 1 tablespoon finely chopped fresh coriander
- 1 tablespoon finely chopped fresh basil
- 1 teaspoon salt

PREP TIME
15 MINUTES

COOK TIME
80 MINUTES

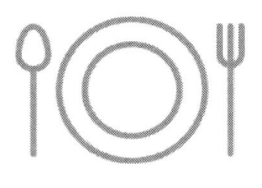

SERVES
10

DIRECTIONS

1. Preheat the oven to 400 °F.
2. In a pan, add oil and zucchini. Sauté until brown, about 10 minutes.
3. Add broth and wine. Simmer on low for about 15 minutes. Add salt.
4. Pour the zucchini and liquid into a blender. Add the herbs and blend until smooth.
5. Spread the diced vegetables on an 8"x8" baking dish. Cover the vegetables with the sauce evenly.
6. Bake uncovered for 50-60 minutes until cooked through. Let it sit for 10-15 minutes before serving.

POULTRY

CHINESE FRIED RICE

INGREDIENTS

2 cups leftover white rice

1 cup cooked chicken breast, shredded

1 egg, beaten

2 tablespoons sesame oil

2 tablespoons soy sauce/coconut amino

1 tablespoon water

PREP TIME
5 MINUTES

COOK TIME
10 MINUTES

DIRECTIONS

1. In a small bowl, combine egg and water.

2. Add 1/2 tablespoon oil to a skillet. Heat over medium heat, add egg and cook undisturbed for 1 minutes. Flip and cook for another 1 minutes. Set aside and cut into shreds.

3. Add the rest of the oil in the skillet. Sauté the chicken for 2 minutes over medium-high heat. Add the rice and stir fry until the grains are not stuck together. Add soy sauce and egg.

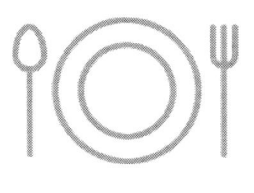

SERVES
4

POULTRY
AVOCADO CHICKEN ZOODLE

PREP TIME
15 MINUTES

COOK TIME
10 MINUTES

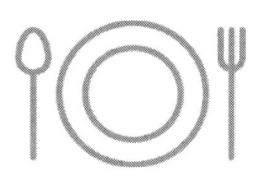

SERVES
4

INGREDIENTS

4 skinless chicken breasts, cut into bite-sized pieces

3 medium zucchini, spiralized

1 medium avocado, seeded, peeled and diced

1/3 cup avocado oil

2 tablespoons apple cider vinegar

2 teaspoons lemon juice

1 teaspoon soy sauce/coconut amino

1 teaspoon salt

1/2 teaspoon ground ginger

DIRECTIONS

1. Use a food processor or blender to combine 2/3 of the oil, 1/2 teaspoon salt, vinegar, lemon juice, soy sauce and ginger.

2. In a skillet, add 1 tablespoon oil and brown the chicken breasts, about 5-7 minutes. Add to the sauce mixture, followed by the diced avocado.

3. Stir fry the zucchini for 1-2 minutes. Pour the chicken and sauce over the zoodle and serve.

POULTRY

CHICKEN PICCATA

INGREDENTS

4 skinless chicken breasts

1 1/2 cups chicken broth, preferably homemade

2 lemons, juice only

1/4 cup chopped fresh parsley

2 tablespoons coconut oil

2 tablespoons coconut cream

Salt to taste

PREP TIME
5 MINUTES

COOK TIME
20 MINUTES

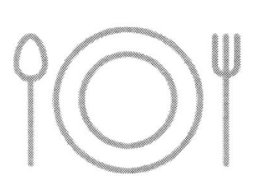

SERVES
4

DIRECTIONS

1. In an oven-proof skillet, add oil. Brown the chicken breasts, about 3 minutes per side. Season with salt. Let it cool and cut into chunks.

2. Add the rest of the ingredients. Bring to a boil and then reduce to low. Simmer for 10 minutes.

3. Add chicken and heat until thoroughly hot.

POULTRY
CREAMY CILANTRO AND LIME CHICKEN

PREP TIME
5 MINUTES

COOK TIME
25 MINUTES

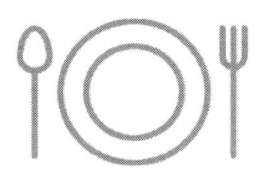

SERVES
4

INGREDENTS

4 skinless chicken breasts

1 cup chicken broth, preferably homemade

1/4 cup coconut cream

3 tablespoons extra virgin olive oil

1 tablespoon chopped fresh cilantro

1 tablespoon lime juice

1/2 teaspoon ground ginger

1/4 teaspoon salt

DIRECTIONS

1. Preheat the oven to 375 °F.

2. In an oven-proof skillet, add 1 tablespoon of olive oil. Brown the chicken breast, about 3 minutes per side. Set aside.

3. Add broth, lime juice, cilantro and ginger. Bring it to a boil and then reduce to low heat. Simmer for 10 minutes.

4. Add coconut cream and the remaining oil. Stir until well combined.

5. Return chicken to the skillet. Bake for 5-10 minutes or until chicken is cooked through.

POULTRY
INDONESIAN PEANUT COCONUT CHICKEN

INGREDENTS

4 skinless chicken breasts, cut into bite-sized pieces

1 13.5-ounce can coconut milk

1/4 cup smooth peanut butter

1 tablespoon coconut oil

1 1/2 teaspoons minced ginger

1 teaspoon maple syrup

1 teaspoon salt

PREP TIME
5 MINUTES

COOK TIME
30 MINUTES

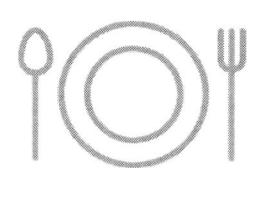

SERVES
4

DIRECTIONS

1. In a medium bowl, combine coconut milk, peanut butter and ginger.

2. In a skillet, add oil and brown the chicken breast, about 5-7 minutes.

3. Add the mixture. Bring to a boil and then reduce to low heat. Simmer for 20 minutes. Season with salt and serve.

POULTRY
HERB ROASTED CHICKEN

INGREDIENTS

1 whole chicken, cut into large pieces

1/4 cup chicken broth

1/4 cup lemon juice

2 tablespoons extra virgin olive oil

2 teaspoons minced fresh rosemary

1 teaspoon minced fresh thyme

1/2 teaspoon finely grated lemon zest

PREP TIME
15 MINUTES

COOK TIME
40 MINUTES

SERVES
4

DIRECTIONS

1. Preheat the oven to 400 °F.

2. In a large bowl, mix all the ingredients. Set aside and marinate for 15 minutes.

3. Place the chicken on a baking dish and pour the marinade on top. Roast for 40 minutes or until cooked through.

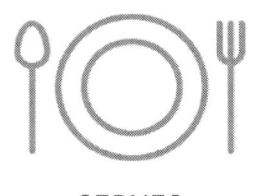

POULTRY
SPAGHETTI SQUASH TURKEY ALFREDO

INGREDENTS

1 small spaghetti squash, halved

1 pound extra-lean ground turkey

1 13.5-ounce can coconut milk

1 medium zucchini, peeled and diced

1/4 cup nutritional yeast (omit if can't tolerate)

2 tablespoons extra virgin olive oil

1 teaspoon salt

PREP TIME
60 MINUTES

COOK TIME
20 MINUTES

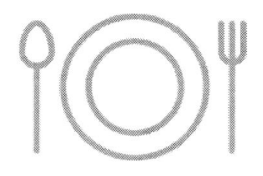

SERVES
4

DIRECTIONS

1. Preheat the oven to 425 °F.

2. Put the spaghetti squash face down on a baking dish. Bake for 45 minutes. Remove the seeds and scrape out the flesh into a large bowl.

3. In a large skillet, brown the ground turkey. Set aside.

4. Sauté zucchini for 5 minutes. Then add coconut milk, yeast and season with salt. Stir until combined. Add the turkey and squash. Heat for another 1-2 minutes and serve.

POULTRY

HARIYALI CHICKEN TIKKA

PREP TIME
120 MINUTES

COOK TIME
20 MINUTES

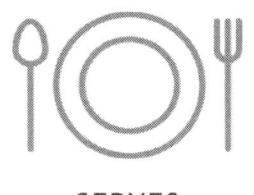

SERVES
4

INGREDIENTS

4 skinless chicken breasts, cut into bite-sized pieces

1 cup chopped fresh cilantro

1/2 cup chopped fresh mint

1 tablespoon grated fresh ginger

1 tablespoon lemon juice

2 teaspoons salt

DIRECTIONS

1. Use a blender or food processor to combine all ingredients except chicken.

2. In a large bowl, mix sauce with chicken thoroughly. Refrigerate for 2 hours to marinate.

3. Preheat the broiler. Line the chicken on a baking dish. Broil for 15-20 minutes or until chicken is cooked through.

POULTRY
SIMPLE TERIYAKI CHICKEN

INGREDIENTS

4 skinless chicken breasts, cut into bite-size

1 1/2 cup no-sugar-added pineapple juice

1/2 cup soy sauce/coconut amino

1 teaspoon ground ginger

PREP TIME
120 MINUTES

COOK TIME
20 MINUTES

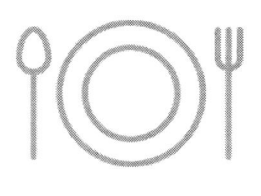

SERVES
4

DIRECTIONS

1. In a large bowl, mix pineapple juice, soy sauce and ginger with chicken thoroughly. Refrigerate for 2 hours to marinate.

2. Preheat the broiler. Line the chicken on a baking dish. Broil for 15-20 minutes or until chicken is cooked through.

POULTRY
APPLE LEMON CHICKEN

INGREDIENTS

4 skinless chicken breasts, cut into bite-sized pieces

2 cups no-sugar-added apple juice

2 lemons, juice only

2 teaspoons chicken bouillon granules

PREP TIME
120 MINUTES

COOK TIME
20 MINUTES

SERVES
4

DIRECTIONS

1. In large bowl, mix apple juice, lemon juice and chicken bouillon granules. Stir until granules dissolve.

2. Mix sauce with chicken thoroughly. Refrigerate for 2 hours to marinate.

3. Preheat the broiler. Line the chicken on a baking dish. Broil for 15-20 minutes or until chicken is cooked through.

POULTRY

CHICKEN BIRYANI

INGREDENTS

- 4 skinless chicken breasts, cut into bite-sized pieces
- 1 cup coconut milk
- 1 cinnamon stick
- 1/2 bunch coriander leaves, chopped
- 1 tablespoon grated fresh ginger
- 1 tablespoon lemon juice
- 1 tablespoon garam masala
- 1/2 teaspoon turmeric
- 1/2 teaspoon cumin powder
- Salt to taste

PREP TIME
120 MINUTES

COOK TIME
20 MINUTES

SERVES
4

DIRECTIONS

1. In a large bowl, combine all ingredients except chicken. Season with salt to taste.
2. Mix sauce with chicken thoroughly. Refrigerate for 2 hours to marinate.
3. Preheat the broiler. Line the chicken on a baking dish. Pour the marinade on top. Broil for 15-20 minutes or until chicken is cooked through.

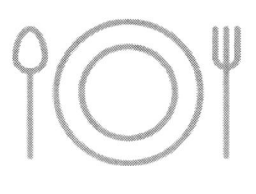

POULTRY
CHICKEN SCHAWARMA

PREP TIME
120 MINUTES

COOK TIME
20 MINUTES

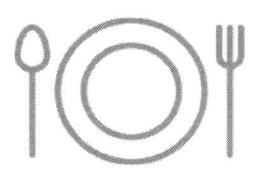

SERVES
4

INGREDENTS

4 skinless chicken breasts, cut into bite-sized pieces

1/4 cup avocado oil

2 teaspoons ground ginger

1 teaspoon salt

3/4 teaspoon turmeric

1/4 teaspoon cinnamon

DIRECTIONS

1. In a large bowl, combine all ingredients except chicken. Season with salt to taste.

2. Mix sauce with chicken thoroughly. Refrigerate for 2 hours to marinate.

3. Preheat the broiler. Line the chicken on a baking dish. Pour the marinade on top. Broil for 15-20 minutes or until chicken is cooked through.

FISH

SIMPLE SALMON CAKE

INGREDIENTS

1 6-ounce can wild caught salmon, drained

1/2 cup pumpkin puree

1/2 tablespoon coconut flour

1/2 tablespoon chopped fresh dill

1/2 tablespoon chopped fresh dill

1 teaspoon coconut oil, not melted

1/4 teaspoon lemon juice

1/4 teaspoon salt

Fat-free cooking spray

PREP TIME
10 MINUTES

COOK TIME
10 MINUTES

SERVES
3

DIRECTIONS

1. In a mixing bowl, combine all ingredients.
2. Divide the mixture into 3 patties or 6 mini patties.
3. Over medium-high heat, pan fry the patties for 2-3 minutes on each side. Flip carefully.

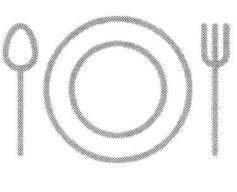

FISH
MACKEREL WITH HERB SAUCE

INGREDIENTS

6 mackerel, cut into fillets

1 cup extra virgin olive oil

1 cup fresh parsley

1/4 cup fresh basil leaves

1 teaspoon apple cider vinegar

Salt to taste

PREP TIME
10 MINUTES

COOK TIME
10 MINUTES

SERVES
3

DIRECTIONS

1. Preheat the oven to 375 °F. Rub 2 tablespoons oil on the fillets. Season with salt and bake for 10 minutes.

2. Meanwhile, use a blender or food processor to blend the rest of the ingredients until smooth.

3. Spoon the herb sauce onto the fillets and serve.

FISH
SALMON IN CREAMED SPINACH

INGREDENTS

4 wild caught salmon fillets, 4-6 ounces each

2 13.5-ounce cans coconut milk

1 large bunch spinach

1/2 cup chopped fresh dill

1/4 cup chopped fresh parsley

2 tablespoons extra virgin olive oil

1 tablespoon lemon juice

1 teaspoon salt

PREP TIME
10 MINUTES

COOK TIME
15 MINUTES

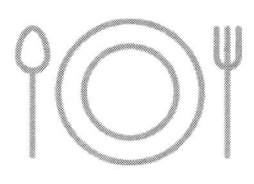

SERVES
4

DIRECTIONS

1. Broil the salmon for about 5 minutes. Break into chunks and set aside to cool.

2. In a sauce pan, add all ingredients except lemon juice. Cook over medium heat until spinach is soft, about 8-10 minutes. Stir in lemon juice.

3. Use a food processor or blender to blend the sauce in small batches.

4. Transfer the creamed spinach to 4 serving bowls. Top with salmon chunks and serve.

FISH

CREAMY TURMERIC COD

PREP TIME
5 MINUTES

COOK TIME
20 MINUTES

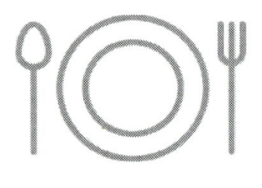

SERVES
3

INGREDIENTS

3 cod fillets

1/2 cup coconut milk

1/2 teaspoon ground turmeric

2 tablespoons chopped fresh parsley

1/2 teaspoon salt

DIRECTIONS

1. Preheat the oven to 350 °F.

2. In a small bowl, combine coconut milk, turmeric and salt.

3. Line the cod fillets on a baking dish. Pour the coconut mixture onto the fillets and sprinkle with parsley. Bake for 15-20 minutes or until cod is cooked through.

FISH
LIME AND GINGER SALMON

INGREDIENTS

2 wild caught salmon fillets, 4-6 ounces each

1 1/2 limes, juice only

1/4 cup water

2 tablespoons minced fresh ginger

2 tablespoons maple syrup

1 tablespoon fish sauce

1 teaspoon coconut oil

1/2 teaspoon salt

PREP TIME
15 MINUTES

COOK TIME
15 MINUTES

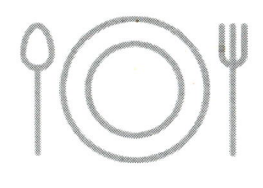

SERVES
2

DIRECTIONS

1. In a small bowl, combine water, maple syrup, lime juice, ginger and fish sauce.
2. Dry the salmon with a towel. Season with salt.
3. Add oil in a skillet. Heat on high until sizzling. Add salmon (skin-side down) and reduce to medium heat. Cook undisturbed until opaque half way up, about 5 minutes. Flip and cook the other side for another 3-4 minutes. Transfer to a serving dish.
4. Serve with steamed vegetables and rice if desired.
5. Add sauce to the pan and cook on medium until thick. Spoon the sauce onto the salmon.

FISH
HERBES DE PROVENCE SALMON ZOODLE

PREP TIME
15 MINUTES

COOK TIME
15 MINUTES

SERVES
3

INGREDIENTS

1 pound wild caught salmon, skin removed and cut into chunks

2 medium zucchini, spiralized

2 medium carrots, peeled and julienned

1 tablespoon lemon juice

2 teaspoons Herbes de Provence (make sure there's no black pepper if can't tolerate)

1 teaspoon salt divided

DIRECTIONS

1. In a large bowl, toss zucchini with 1 tablespoon oil. Set aside.

2. In a large skillet, add the remaining oil and Herbes de Provence. Cook until fragrant over medium heat. Add the carrot and cook for another 5 minutes.

3. Move the carrot to the side. Add the salmon. Season with half of the salt. Cover and cook for 5 minutes, flipping once halfway through.

4. Add the zoodle on top. Sprinkle the remaining salt. Cover and cook for another 3 minutes.

5. Add the lemon juice, mix well and serve.

FISH
BAKED COD WITH ZUCCHINI

INGREDIENTS

4 cod fillets, 4-6 ounces each

3 medium zucchini, peeled and diced

1 lemon, sliced

2 tablespoons extra virgin olive oil, divided

1 tablespoon chopped fresh dill

1/2 tablespoon salt

PREP TIME
15 MINUTES

COOK TIME
20 MINUTES

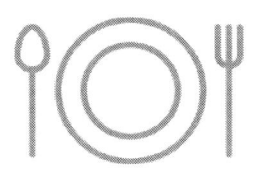

SERVES
4

DIRECTIONS

1. Preheat the oven to 350 °F.

2. Rub 1 tablespoon of oil on cod fillets. Line the fillets on a baking dish, season with salt, sprinkle with dills and top with lemon slices.

3. In a skillet, add the remaining oil and zucchini, sauté for 5 minutes. Then add the zucchini on top of the fish.

4. Bake for 10-15 minutes or until fish is cooked through.

FISH
SWEET AND SOUR GLAZED SALMON

PREP TIME
10 MINUTES

COOK TIME
25 MINUTES

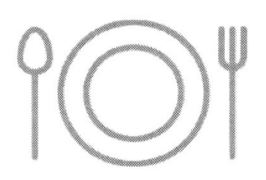

SERVES
4

INGREDENTS

4 wild caught salmon fillets, 4-6 ounces each

1 cup pineapple chunks

1 tablespoon extra virgin olive oil

1 tablespoon maple syrup

1 tablespoon lemon juice

1 teaspoon salt

DIRECTIONS

1. Preheat the oven to 400 °F.

2. Rub oil over the fillet. Season the salmon with salt. Line the fillets in a baking dish. Top with pineapple chunks. Bake for 20 minutes.

3. Meanwhile, combine maple syrup and lemon juice in a small bowl.

4. Move the pineapple aside. Then spread the glaze over the salmon fillet. Broil for another 5 minutes before serving.

FISH
FRENCH SALT COD BRANDADE

INGREDIENTS

1 pound salt cod, salt rinsed off and immersed in filtered water overnight

1/2 pound rutabaga, peeled and cut into 1-inch wedges

1 cup extra virgin olive oil

1/2 cup coconut cream

2 tablespoons chopped fresh parsley

3 sprigs thyme

1 bay leaf

1 teaspoon salt

PREP TIME
10 MINUTES

COOK TIME
60 MINUTES

SERVES
4

DIRECTIONS

1. Preheat the oven to 350 °F.

2. Toast the rutabaga with 1/4 cup oil. Season with salt. Bake for 40-45 minutes until cooked through. Mash and set aside.

3. Meanwhile, in a skillet, add cod, thyme, bay leaf and cover with unsalted water. Bring to a boil and then reduce to low. Simmer for 10 minutes. Discard the water, thyme and bay leaf.

4. Break cod into chunks. Remove bones and skin. Add the chunks to a stand mixer with paddle. Slowly add the remaining oil while mixing over medium speed, followed by coconut cream and rutabaga mash.

5. Transfer to a baking dish and bake for 10-15 minutes, or until brown on top.

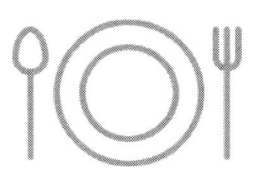

FISH
CITRUS AND SAGE SALMON

INGREDIENTS

4 wild caught salmon fillets, 4-6 ounces each

1 small orange, washed

1 lemon, washed

2 tablespoons chopped fresh sage

2 tablespoons extra virgin olive oil

1 tablespoon maple syrup

1 teaspoon salt

PREP TIME
60 MINUTES

COOK TIME
15 MINUTES

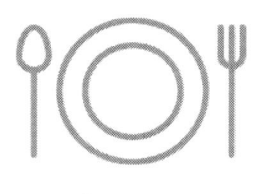

SERVES
4

DIRECTIONS

1. In a mixing bowl, zest lemon and orange. Squeeze the juice of 1/2 lemon and 1/2 orange. Add oil, maple syrup and salt. Stir until combined.

2. Dry the salmon fillets with a paper towel. Add to the mixing bowl. Spread sauce over the fillets. Refrigerate and marinate for 60 minutes.

3. Preheat the oven to 400 °F by the last 15 minutes. Cut the remaining orange and lemon into thin slices.

4. Place the salmon fillets in a baking dish, top with sage, lemon and orange slices. Bake for 13-15 minutes.

FISH

GEFILTE FISH

INGREDENTS

1 pound halibut fillets, cut into small chunks

1/2 pound salmon fillets, cut into small chunks

3 medium carrots, peeled and grated

2 large eggs

1/2 cup chopped fresh parsley

1/4 cup chopped fresh dill

2 tablespoons extra virgin olive oil

1 tablespoon lemon juice

1 teaspoon salt

PREP TIME
120 MINUTES

COOK TIME
20 MINUTES

SERVES
8

DIRECTIONS

1. Use a food processor to pulse the fish until finely ground. Add the rest of the ingredients until combined. Refrigerate the mixture for 2 hours.

2. Prepare a pot of water and bring it to a boil. Scoop spoonful of the mixture. Shape into balls and put into boiling water. Cook for 15-20 minutes.

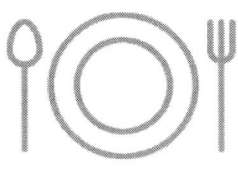

DESSERT & SNACK
ROASTED BUTTERNUT SQUASH HUMMUS

PREP TIME
5 MINUTES

COOK TIME
NA

SERVES
6

INGREDIENTS

1 small Butternut Squash, peeled, seeded, and cut into 1-inch cubes

2 tablespoons fresh lemon juice

2 tablespoons extra virgin olive oil

1/4 cup tahini (omit if can't tolerate)

1/4 cup chopped fresh parsley

1 tablespoon chopped fresh dill

1 tablespoon chopped fresh coriander

1/2 teaspoon salt

1/2 teaspoon cumin

DIRECTIONS

1. Toss squash, oil, herbs and salt together. Spread evenly on a baking dish. Bake for 20-25 minutes or until squash is tender.

2. Transfer to a food processor. Add the rest of the ingredients and blend until smooth.

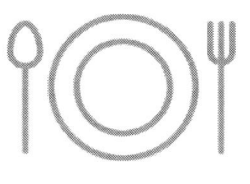

DESSERT & SNACK
ALMOND BUTTER ICE CREAM

INGREDIENTS

- 2 very ripe frozen bananas
- 2 tablespoons unsalted creamy almond butter
- 1/4 teaspoon salt

PREP TIME
5 MINUTES

COOK TIME
NA

SERVES
2

DIRECTIONS

1. Add banana, almond butter and salt to a food processor. Blend on low to medium speed until creamy and smooth.

DESSERT & SNACK
WILD SALMON PATÉ

PREP TIME
5 MINUTES

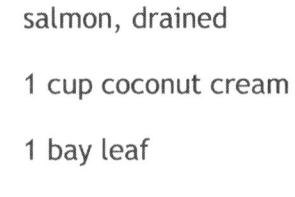

COOK TIME
NA

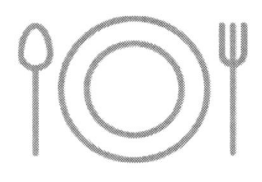

SERVES
16

INGREDIENTS

2 6-ounce cans wild caught salmon, drained

1 cup coconut cream

1 bay leaf

2 tablespoons lemon juice

1 tablespoon chopped fresh parsley

1 tablespoon chopped fresh chives

1 tablespoon chopped fresh dill

3/4 teaspoon salt

DIRECTIONS

1. Use a food processor/blender to blend all ingredients until well combined.

DESSERT & SNACK
CINNAMON COCONUT PUDDING

INGREDENTS

1 13.5-ounce can coconut milk

3/4 tablespoon gelatin

1/2 teaspoon vanilla extract

1/2 teaspoon cinnamon

2 tablespoon maple syrup

PREP TIME
5 MINUTES

COOK TIME
5 MINUTES

DIRECTIONS

1. In a sauce pan, add all ingredients except cinnamon. Heat on low until well combined. Remove from heat.

2. Sprinkle the gelatin on top and stir until dissolved. Reheat if necessary.

3. Pour the mixture into 4 pudding cups. Let it cool at room temperature before refrigerating for a few hours until the pudding is set.

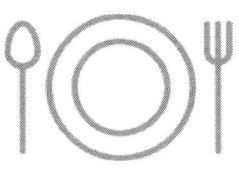

SERVES
4

DESSERT & SNACK
SPAGHETTI SQUASH HASH BROWN

PREP TIME
5 MINUTES

COOK TIME
20 MINUTES

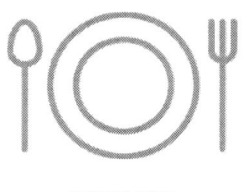

SERVES
2

INGREDENTS

2 cups cooked and shredded spaghetti squash

1 tablespoon extra virgin olive oil

1 teaspoon chopped sage

Pinch of rosemary

Pinch of salt

DIRECTIONS

1. In a mixing bowl, combine squash, herbs and salt.

2. Divide the mixture into 4 portions and mold into patties. Use a paper towel to absorb the extra moisture.

3. Pan fry for 6-8 minutes per side or until golden brown.

DESSERT & SNACK
MINI PUMPKIN BANANA PIE

INGREDENTS

1 1/2 cups pumpkin puree

2 very ripe medium bananas

1/4 cup maple syrup

1 teaspoon cinnamon

1/4 teaspoon ground ginger

1/4 teaspoon nutmeg

1/4 teaspoon salt

PREP TIME
5 MINUTES

COOK TIME
25 MINUTES

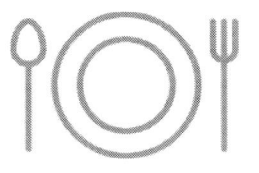

DIRECTIONS

1. Preheat the oven to 350 °F.

2. Blend all ingredients in a blender/food processor until smooth.

3. Divide the mixture into 12 baking cups. Bake for 20-25 minutes until cooked through.

SERVES
12

DESSERT & SNACK
COCONUT RICE PUDDING

PREP TIME
5 MINUTES

COOK TIME
30 MINUTES

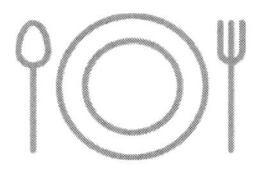

SERVES
6

INGREDIENTS

1 13.5-ounce can coconut milk

1 cup uncooked white rice, rinsed and drained

1 cup unsweetened almond milk

1/4 cup maple syrup

1 1/2 teaspoons vanilla extract

1 1/2 teaspoons cinnamon

Pinch of sea salt

Shredded coconut, for topping (optional)

DIRECTIONS

1. In a sauce pan, add coconut milk and bring it to a boil. Add rice. Heat until boiling then reduce to low. Cover and simmer for 20 minutes.

2. Remove lid and add the rest of the ingredients except shredded coconut. Cook for another 8-10 minutes while stirring.

3. Pour the mixture in a container. Let it cool at room temperature. Refrigerate for 90 minutes before serving.

DESSERT & SNACK
RICE CRACKERS WITH HERBS

INGREDENTS

2 cups cooked white rice

6 basil leaves, chopped

2 tablespoons chopped fresh parsley

1 teaspoon fresh rosemary

Salt to taste

PREP TIME
5 MINUTES

COOK TIME
35 MINUTES

DIRECTIONS

1. Preheat the oven to 350 °F.

2. Use a food processor/blender to blend all ingredients until well combined.

3. Use a tablespoon to scoop out the mixture. Press/roll into flat crackers, about 1 1/2-inch in diameter.

4. Bake for 20-25 minutes.

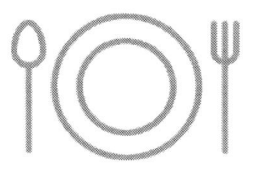

SERVES
8

DESSERT & SNACK
APPLE COCONUT BUTTER CUP

INGREDIENTS

1 medium apple, peeled, cored and diced

1/2 cup coconut manna/coconut butter

2 tablespoons coconut oil

2 tablespoons almond butter

1 teaspoon vanilla extract

2 teaspoons cinnamon

Pinch of salt

PREP TIME
5 MINUTES

COOK TIME
45 MINUTES

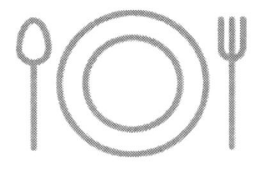

SERVES
12

DIRECTIONS

1. In a sauce pan, add oil and apple. Cook until soft, about 8-10 minutes. Remove from heat. Stir in coconut butter, cinnamon and salt and mix until well combined.

2. Spread 1/2 teaspoon almond butter in the bottom of each baking cup. Top with the apple mixture.

3. Freeze for 30 minutes before serving.

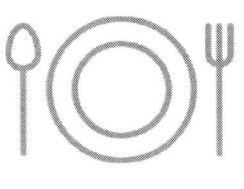

DESSERT & SNACK
BANANA COCONUT ICE CREAM

INGREDENTS

4 very ripe frozen bananas, thawed

2 13.5-ounce cans coconut milk

1 cup maple syrup

1 tablespoon vanilla extract

PREP TIME
5 MINUTES

COOK TIME
45 MINUTES

SERVES
6

DIRECTIONS

1. Blend all ingredients in a blender/food processor until smooth.

2. Add to ice cream maker and prepare according to manufacturers' instruction

DESSERT & SNACK
CARROT COCONUT TRUFFLES

PREP TIME
10 MINUTES

COOK TIME
50 MINUTES

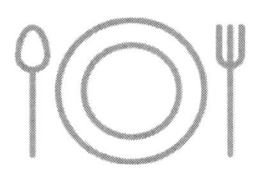

SERVES
12

INGREDENTS

4 medium carrots, peeled and quartered lengthwise

1/2 cup coconut butter

1/4 cup shredded coconut

1 tablespoon coconut oil

1 tablespoon cinnamon

1 teaspoon vanilla extract

1 teaspoon ground ginger

1/4 teaspoon salt

DIRECTIONS

1. Preheat the oven to 400 °F.

2. In a baking dish, toss carrots with coconut oil and bake for 20-25 minutes or until tender. Set aside to cool for 10-15 minutes.

3. Meanwhile, mix the shredded coconut with salt and spread it on a plate.

4. Use a food processor/blender to blend carrots, coconut butter, cinnamon, vanilla and ginger until well combined.

5. Use a tablespoon to scoop out the mixture. Mold into truffles and roll in the shredded coconut. Refrigerate

DESSERT & SNACK
COCONUT PLANTAIN MACARON

INGREDENTS

1 yellow plantain

1 1/4 cup shredded coconut

1 tablespoon extra virgin olive oil

1/4 cup maple syrup

3 teaspoon cinnamon

PREP TIME
15 MINUTES

COOK TIME
45 MINUTES

SERVES
9

DIRECTIONS

1. Preheat the oven to 400 °F.
2. Blend all ingredients except coconut in a blender/food processor until smooth.
3. In a mixing bowl, stir in the coconut and the mixture.
4. Scoop out 1/4 cup of mixture and roll into balls.
5. Bake for 25-30 minutes or until golden brown

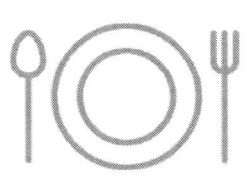

Slow Cooker Recipes

BREAKFAST 83-88

SOUPS & BROTHS 89-93

SIDE DISH 94-96

DESSERT 97-104

CHICKEN 105 - 120

BEEF, LAMB AND PORK 121 - 132

SLOW COOKER
OAT-STUFFED APPLES

INGREDIENTS

6 green apples, top cut off and cored, leaving bottom intact

1 cup oats

1/4 cup nut butter

2 tablespoons raw honey

1 tablespoon coconut oil

1 teaspoon cinnamon

1 teaspoon nutmeg

PREP TIME
5 MINUTES

COOK TIME
2 HOURS

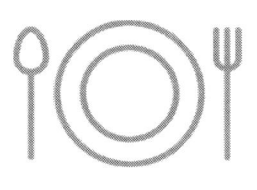

SERVES
6

DIRECTIONS

1. In a medium bowl, combine all ingredients except apples.
2. Stuff apples and put into slow cooker.
3. Cook on low for 2 hours.

SLOW COOKER PUMPKIN PIE OATMEAL

PREP TIME
10 MINUTES

COOK TIME
8 HOURS

SERVES
4

INGREDIENTS

1 cup pumpkin puree

1 cup oats

2 cups water

2 cups coconut milk or almond milk

2 tablespoons maple syrup

1 teaspoon vanilla extract

1 teaspoon pumpkin pie spice

1/2 teaspoon cinnamon

1/4 teaspoon salt

DIRECTIONS

1. Mix all ingredients in the slow cooker.
2. Cook on low for 8 hours.
3. Top with desired toppings and serve.

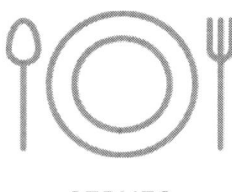

SLOW COOKER
CHINESE CHICKEN CONGEE

INGREDIENTS

1 cup white rice, rinsed

7 cups water

1 cup chicken broth

2 bone-in chicken thighs

1-inch fresh ginger roots, peeled and sliced

Soy sauce or coconut amino for serving

PREP TIME
10 MINUTES

COOK TIME
8 HOURS

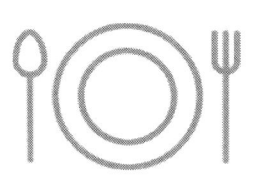

SERVES
4

DIRECTIONS

1. Mix all ingredients in the slow cooker.
2. Cook on low for 8 hours.
3. Remove chicken skin and shred meat. Serve with soy sauce/coconut amino if desired.

SLOW COOKER
BUTTERNUT SQUASH APPLE OATMEAL

PREP TIME
10 MINUTES

COOK TIME
8 HOURS

SERVES
4

INGREDENTS

1 medium butternut squash, peeled and cubed

2 medium apples, peeled, cored and diced

1 cup coconut milk

3/4 cup almond flour (omit if can't tolerate)

1/4 cup nut butter of your choice

1 tablespoon maple syrup

1 teaspoon cinnamon

1/2 teaspoon nutmeg

Toppings of your choice

DIRECTIONS

1. Mix all ingredients in the slow cooker.
2. Cook on low for 8 hours.
3. Use an immersion blender or potato masher to mash into desired consistency.
4. Top with desired toppings and serve.

SLOW COOKER
TURKEY BREAKFAST CASSEROLE

INGREDIENTS

- 1 pound lean ground turkey
- 1 small butternut squash, peeled, seeded and sliced
- 12 eggs, beaten
- 3 cups spinach
- 1 cup coconut milk
- 1 tablespoon coconut oil
- 1 teaspoon sage
- 1/4 teaspoon salt

PREP TIME 10 MINUTES

COOK TIME 8 HOURS

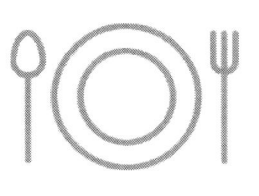

SERVES 6

DIRECTIONS

1. Season the meat with sage and salt. Whisk eggs with coconut milk
2. Grease the slow cooker with coconut oil. Add squash, followed by meat, egg mixture and spinach.
3. Cook on low for 8 hours.

SLOW COOKER
PEANUT BUTTER BREAKFAST BAR

PREP TIME
10 MINUTES

COOK TIME
8 HOURS

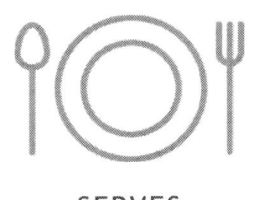

SERVES
14

INGREDIENTS

3/4 cup mashed bananas

2 large eggs

1 cup oats

1 1/2 cups coconut milk or almond milk

3 tablespoons smooth peanut butter

3 tablespoons honey

DIRECTIONS

1. Microwave peanut butter and honey for 30 seconds. Combine with almond milk, banana and cinnamon. Add eggs and mix well. Stir in oats and transfer the mixture to the greased slow cooker.

2. Cook on low for 8 hours.

SLOW COOKER
GREEK CHICKEN SOUP

INGREDIENTS

1 pound bone-in skinless chicken breast

3 eggs

2 stalk celery, roughly chopped

4 cups chicken broth

2 cups water

1/4 cup lemon juice

1/2 cup uncooked white rice, rinsed and drained

1 teaspoon salt

PREP TIME
10 MINUTES

COOK TIME
6 HOURS

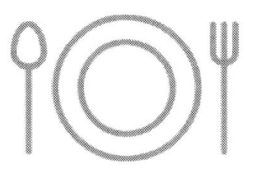

SERVES
6

DIRECTIONS

1. Place chicken, celery, rice, broth, water and salt in the slow cooker

2. Cook on low for 6 hours.

3. Remove celery if can't tolerate. Shred meat and discard the bones.

4. In a medium bowl, whisk eggs with lemon juice. Spoon out a few tablespoons of hot broth and slowly stir into the lemon mixture. Then add the mixture to the soup and stir until combined.

SLOW COOKER
CLASSIC CHICKEN AND RICE SOUP

INGREDENTS

PREP TIME
10 MINUTES

2 pound bone-in skinless chicken breast

4 medium carrots, peeled and chopped

10 cups chicken broth

1 cup uncooked white rice, rinsed and drained

2 bay leaves

1/2 teaspoon dried thyme

1/2 tablespoon salt

COOK TIME
6 HOURS

DIRECTIONS

1. Mix all ingredients in the slow cooker.
2. Cook on low for 6 hours.
3. Shred meat, discard the bones and bay leaves. Adjust seasoning if needed.

SERVES
8

SLOW COOKER
LEMONY KALE CHICKEN SOUP

INGREDENTS

1 pound bone-in skinless chicken breast

6 cups chicken broth

1/2 cup olive oil

1 bunch kale, roughly chopped

Zest of 3 lemons

2 tablespoons lemon juice

salt to taste

PREP TIME
10 MINUTES

COOK TIME
6 HOURS

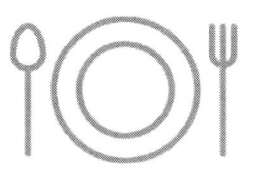

SERVES
6

DIRECTIONS

1. Use a blender to blend 2 cups of broth with olive oil until it emulsifies.
2. Mix all ingredients in the slow cooker.
3. Cook on low for 6 hours.
4. Shred meat and serve.

SLOW COOKER
CURRY PUMPKIN CARROT SOUP

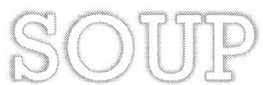

PREP TIME
10 MINUTES

COOK TIME
8 HOURS

SERVES
6

INGREDIENTS

7 medium carrots, peeled and cut into chunks

12 ounces pumpkin, peeled, seeded and cut into chunks

4 cups chicken broth

3/4 teaspoon turmeric

1/2 teaspoon salt

1/2 teaspoon cinnamon

1/4 teaspoon ground ginger

DIRECTIONS

1. Mix all ingredients in the slow cooker.
2. Cook on low for 8 hours.
3. Use an immersion blender to blend into desired consistency.

SLOW COOKER
TURMERIC BONE BROTH

INGREDIENTS

- 1 whole chicken carcass
- 4 stalks celery, roughly chopped
- 2 medium carrot, peeled and roughly chopped
- 2 medium onions, quartered
- 2 sprigs thyme
- 2 bay leaves
- 2 teaspoons turmeric
- 1 tablespoon salt
- 1 tablespoon apple cider vinegar

PREP TIME
10 MINUTES

COOK TIME
8 HOURS

SERVES
20

DIRECTIONS

1. Mix all ingredients in the slow cooker. Add enough water to cover the carcass or about an inch from the top
2. Cook on low for 8-10 hours.
3. Skim off fat from the surface. Strain the bones and vegetables using a strainer.

(The broth can be refrigerated up to a week and freeze for up to 1 month)

SLOW COOKER
THYME BUTTER RICE

PREP TIME
15 MINUTES

COOK TIME
3 HOURS

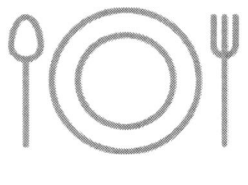

SERVES
4

INGREDIENTS

2 cups medium to long grain white rice

8 ounces or sliced mushrooms

4 cups chicken broth

2 tablespoons butter

1/2 teaspoon dried thyme

1/2 teaspoon oregano

DIRECTIONS

1. In a pan, sauté rice with butter and herbs for 2-4 minutes. Transfer to the slow cooker.

2. Add the remaining ingredients.

3. Cover and cook on low for 2 hours. Stir and check texture. Add more broth if needed and cook for another 30-60 minutes.

SLOW COOKER BUTTERNUT SQUASH RISOTTO

INGREDENTS

1 medium butternut squash, peeled, seeded and cut into 1/4" chunks

1 1/2 cups uncooked short grain white rice

4 cups chicken broth

1/2 teaspoon salt

PREP TIME
15 MINUTES

COOK TIME
5 HOURS

SERVES
8

DIRECTIONS

1. Mix all ingredients in the slow cooker.

2. Cover and cook on low for 4 hours. Stir and check texture. Add more broth if needed and cook for another 30-60 minutes.

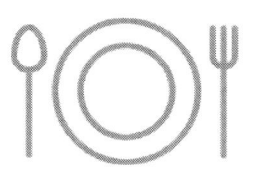

SLOW COOKER
ROSEMARY ACORN SQUASH

PREP TIME
5 MINUTES

COOK TIME
8 HOURS

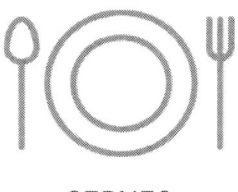

SERVES
8

INGREDIENTS

- 1 medium acorn squash, peeled, seeded and cut into wedges
- 1/2 cup vegetables broth
- 2 tablespoons extra virgin olive oil
- 3 tablespoons chopped fresh rosemary
- 1 tablespoon balsamic vinegar
- 1 teaspoon salt

DIRECTIONS

1. Line the squash wedges in the slow cooker. Add broth. Drizzle with oil and vinegar. Sprinkle with salt and rosemary.
2. Cover and cook on low for 8 hours.

SLOW COOKER
SIMPLE PLANTAIN MASH

INGREDIENTS

6 ripe plantains, peeled and cut into chunks

1 1/2 cups water

1 15-ounce can coconut milk

1/2 cup maple syrup

1/2 cup chopped almonds

1/4 cup butter

1 teaspoon cinnamon

PREP TIME
5 MINUTES

COOK TIME
4 HOURS

DIRECTIONS

1. Mix all ingredients in the slow cooker.
2. Cover and cook on low for 4 hours.
3. Serve with coconut cream if desired.

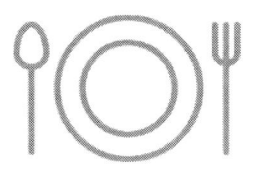

SERVES
6

SLOW COOKER
COCONUT RICE PUDDING

PREP TIME
5 MINUTES

COOK TIME
4 HOURS

SERVES
8

INGREDIENTS

6 cups coconut milk

1 15-ounce can coconut cream

2 cups uncooked white rice

3 tablespoons butter, melted

1 teaspoon cinnamon

1/2 teaspoon vanilla extract

1/4 teaspoon salt

DIRECTIONS

1. Grease the slow cooker with 1 tablespoon butter.
2. Mix all ingredients in the slow cooker.
3. Cover and cook on low for 4 hours, stirring occasionally.

SLOW COOKER PUMPKIN BUTTER

INGREDIENTS

2 15-ounce cans pumpkin puree

1 cup fresh apple juice

1/2 cup maple syrup

2 teaspoons cinnamon

1/2 teaspoon ground ginger

1/2 teaspoon ground cloves

Pinch of salt

PREP TIME
5 MINUTES

COOK TIME
5 HOURS

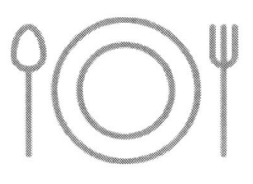

SERVES
16

DIRECTIONS

1. Mix all ingredients in the slow cooker.
2. Cover and cook on low for 5 hours, stirring occasionally. Adjust sweetness if needed

SLOW COOKER BLACKBERRY JAM

PREP TIME
5 MINUTES

COOK TIME
5 HOURS

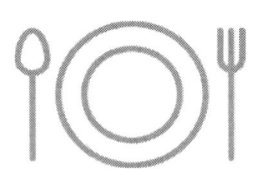

SERVES
16

INGREDENTS

2 pounds fresh blackberries

1/2 cup maple syrup

2 limes, juice only

2 teaspoons ground nutmeg

DIRECTIONS

1. Mix all ingredients in the slow cooker.
2. Cover and cook on low for 4 hours, stirring occasionally.
3. Cook on low, uncovered for another 1 hour until the jam thickened. Let it cool.
4. Use an immersion blender to blend into desired consistency. Adjust sweetness if needed.

SLOW COOKER
CRANBERRY ORANGE SAUCE

INGREDENTS

2 pounds fresh cranberries

1 1/3 cups fresh orange juice

1/2 cup maple syrup

2 tablespoons orange zest

1 teaspoon vanilla extract

PREP TIME
5 MINUTES

COOK TIME
8 HOURS

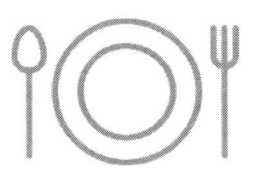

SERVES
16

DIRECTIONS

1. Mix all ingredients in the slow cooker.

2. Cover and cook on low for 8 hours.

3. Adjust sweetness if needed

SLOW COOKER PEAR BUTTER

PREP TIME
5 MINUTES

COOK TIME
8 HOURS

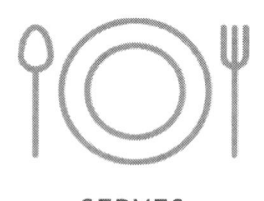

SERVES
16

INGREDIENTS

- 2 pounds pears, peeled, cored, chopped
- 1 cups fresh apple juice
- 1/2 cup maple syrup
- 2 teaspoons cinnamon
- 1/2 teaspoon ground ginger
- 1/2 teaspoon ground nutmeg
- 1/2 teaspoon cardamom

DIRECTIONS

1. Mix all ingredients in the slow cooker.
2. Cover and cook on low for 8 hours. Let it cool.
3. Use an immersion blender to blend into desired consistency. Adjust sweetness if needed.

SLOW COOKER
CLASSIC APPLE SAUCE

INGREDENTS

2 pounds apples, peeled, cored, chopped

1 cups water

1/2 cup maple syrup

1 lemon, juice only

2 teaspoons cinnamon

2/3 teaspoon all spice

2/3 teaspoon clove

2/3 teaspoon ground ginger

Pinch of ground nutmeg

PREP TIME
10 MINUTES

COOK TIME
8 HOURS

SERVES
16

DIRECTIONS

1. Mix all ingredients in the slow cooker.

2. Cover and cook on low for 8 hours. Let it cool.

3. Use an immersion blender to blend into desired consistency. Adjust sweetness if needed.

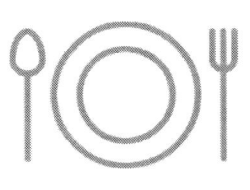

SLOW COOKER
COCONUT YOGURT

PREP TIME
5 MINUTES

COOK TIME
15.5 HOURS

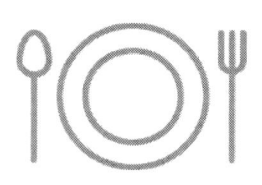

SERVES
8

INGREDENTS

2 15-ounce cans full fat coconut milk

1 tablespoon maple syrup

2 teaspoons gelatin

2 teaspoons probiotic powder

DIRECTIONS

1. Add coconut milk to slow cooker. Sprinkle gelatin on top and let it sit for 5 minutes before whisking it in.

2. Cover and cook on low for 2 1/2 hours. Then turn off the slow cooker and let it sit for 3 hours, covered.

3. Scoop out 1/4 cup coconut milk and mix with probiotic powder. Gently stir in the mixture.

4. Cover and wrap the whole slow cooker with a thick towel. Let it sit for 8 hours.

5. Transfer to a container and refrigerate for at least 6 hours before serving.

SLOW COOKER
LEMON CILANTRO CHICKEN & RICE

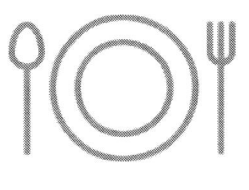

INGREDENTS

1 1/2 pounds chicken thighs

1 cup uncooked white rice

2 1/4 cups chicken broth

1/2 cup chopped fresh cilantro

1/4 cup fresh lemon juice

1 1/2 teaspoon salt

PREP TIME
10 MINUTES

COOK TIME
7 HOURS

SERVES
4

DIRECTIONS

1. Season chicken with salt.
2. Stir together the rest of the ingredients in the slow cooker. Place chicken on top.
3. Cook on low for 6-7 hours.

SLOW COOKER
CHICKEN RICE CASSEROLE

PREP TIME
10 MINUTES

COOK TIME
7 HOURS

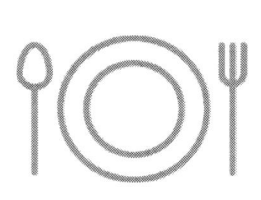

SERVES
6

INGREDENTS

1 1/2 pounds chicken thighs

6 ounces sliced mushrooms

1 cup uncooked white rice

1 cup full fat coconut cream

1 cup chicken broth

1/4 cup water

1 1/2 teaspoon salt

DIRECTIONS

1. Season chicken with salt.
2. Stir together the rest of the ingredients in the slow cooker. Place chicken on top.
3. Cook on low for 6-7 hours.
4. Shred chicken and serve.

SLOW COOKER CHICKEN STROGANOFF

INGREDENTS

1 pound chicken breast

8 ounces sliced mushrooms

1 cup full fat coconut milk

1 cup chicken broth

1 tablespoon chopped fresh parsley

1 1/2 teaspoons dried thyme

1/2 teaspoon salt

PREP TIME
10 MINUTES

COOK TIME
8 HOURS

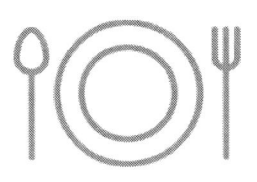

SERVES
4

DIRECTIONS

1. Mix all ingredients in the slow cooker.
2. Cook on low for 6-8 hours.
3. Shred the meat and serve

SLOW COOKER
MOROCCAN CHICKEN DRUMSTICK

PREP TIME
10 MINUTES

COOK TIME
8 HOURS

SERVES
8

INGREDENTS

- 2 pounds chicken drumstick
- 2 cups chicken broth
- 2 large carrots, peeled and diced
- 1 cup dried apricots, chopped
- 1 1/2 tablespoons grated fresh ginger
- 1 1/2 teaspoons sea salt
- 1 teaspoon cumin
- 1 teaspoon turmeric
- 1 teaspoon cinnamon
- 1/2 teaspoon coriander
- 1/2 cardamom powder

DIRECTIONS

5. Mix all ingredients in the slow cooker.
6. Cook on low for 6-8 hours.

SLOW COOKER
PEAR CRANBERRY SQUASH CHICKEN

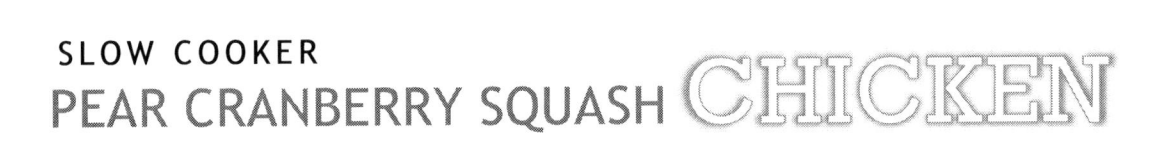

INGREDENTS

- 1 1/2 pounds chicken breast
- 1 medium butternut squash, peeled, seeded and diced
- 1 medium pear, cored and sliced
- 1 cup fresh cranberry
- 1 cup chicken broth
- 2 bay leaves
- 2 teaspoon cinnamon
- 1 teaspoon salt

PREP TIME 10 MINUTES

COOK TIME 8 HOURS

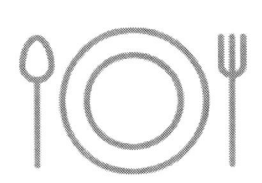

SERVES 6

DIRECTIONS

1. Season the chicken with salt.
2. Layer squash in the bottom of the slow cooker, followed by chicken, pear, cranberry and bay leaves. Sprinkle cinnamon and add broth.
3. Cook on low for 6-8 hours.

SLOW COOKER
MILD CHICKEN CARNITAS

INGREDENTS

1 1/2 pounds chicken breast

1 cup fresh orange juice

1/4 cup fresh lime juice

1 teaspoon ground cumin

1 teaspoon ground oregano

1/2 teaspoon salt

PREP TIME
10 MINUTES

COOK TIME
8 HOURS

SERVES
6

DIRECTIONS

1. Mix all ingredients in the slow cooker.
2. Cook on low for 6-8 hours.
3. Shred the meat and serve

SLOW COOKER
BALSAMIC CHICKEN THIGHS

INGREDIENTS

8 boneless skinless chicken thighs

1/2 cup balsamic vinegar

2 tablespoons extra virgin olive oil

1 teaspoon dried basil

1 teaspoon dried oregano

1 teaspoon dried rosemary

1/2 teaspoon dried thyme

1/2 teaspoon salt

PREP TIME
10 MINUTES

COOK TIME
8 HOURS

SERVES
8

DIRECTIONS

1. Rub the spices and salt over the chicken thighs and place them in the slow cooker. Drizzle with oil and add vinegar.

2. Cook on low for 6-8 hours.

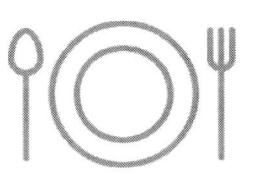

SLOW COOKER
APPLE ACORN SQUASH CHICKEN

PREP TIME
10 MINUTES

COOK TIME
8 HOURS

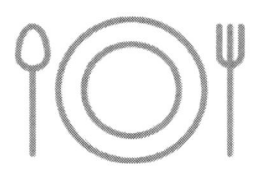

SERVES
12

INGREDIENTS

1 whole chicken, about 4-5 pounds

1 medium acorn squash, peeled, seeded and cut into wedges

3 medium apples, peeled, cored and chopped

1 tablespoon ground cumin

1 tablespoon curry powder (replace with 1/2 tablespoon turmeric if can't tolerate)

2 teaspoons ground coriander

1 teaspoon salt

DIRECTIONS

1. Rub the spices and salt over the chicken.
2. Layer squash in the bottom of the slow cooker, followed by chicken. Top with apple chunks.
3. Cook on low for 6-8 hours.
4. Shred meat, discard bones and serve.

SLOW COOKER LEMON ROSEMARY CHICKEN

INGREDIENTS

1 1/2 pounds chicken breast

1 cup chicken broth

1 lemon, sliced

5 sprigs fresh rosemary

1/4 teaspoon salt

PREP TIME
10 MINUTES

COOK TIME
8 HOURS

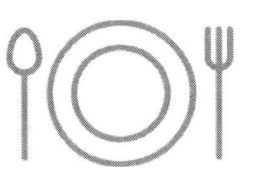

SERVES
6

DIRECTIONS

1. Season chicken with salt and place the chicken in the slow cooker. Top with lemon and rosemary then pour broth over.

2. Cook on low for 6-8 hours.

3. Shred meat and serve.

SLOW COOKER
THAI ROAST CHICKEN

PREP TIME
10 MINUTES

COOK TIME
8 HOURS

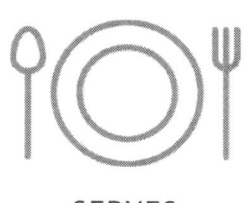

SERVES
8

INGREDIENTS

- 1 whole chicken, about 4-5 pounds
- 2 cups full fat coconut milk
- 3 tablespoons extra virgin olive oil
- 4 fresh sage leaves
- 2 stalks lemongrass, sliced
- 1 cinnamon stick
- 1 lemon, zest only
- 1 teaspoon salt

DIRECTIONS

1. Season chicken with salt. Drizzle with olive oil. Top with lemon grass, sage leaves, cinnamon and lemon zest. Add coconut milk.

2. Cook on low for 6-8 hours.

3. Shred meat, discard bones , lemon grass, cinnamon, sage leaves and serve.

SLOW COOKER
TEYIRAKI CHICKEN

INGREDENTS

2 pounds chicken breast

1/2 cup soy sauce or coconut amino

1/2 cup honey

1/4 cup water

1/4 cup white wine vinegar

3/4 cup ground ginger

PREP TIME
10 MINUTES

COOK TIME
8 HOURS

SERVES
8

DIRECTIONS

1. In a small bowl, combine all seasoning ingredients.
2. Place chicken in slow cooker and pour the mixture over chicken.
3. Cook on low for 6-8 hours.
4. Shred meat and serve.

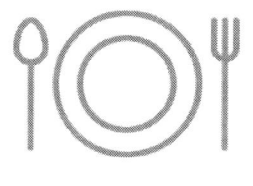

SLOW COOKER
FENNEL ORANGE CHICKEN

PREP TIME
10 MINUTES

COOK TIME
8 HOURS

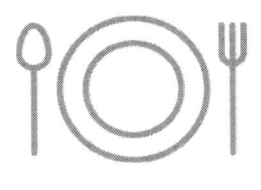

SERVES
6

INGREDENTS

1 1/2 pounds chicken breast

3 large carrots, peeled and diced

1 fennel bulb, cored and thinly sliced

1 orange, thinly sliced

3 tablespoons extra virgin olive oil

1 tablespoons apple cider vinegar

1 teaspoon herbes de provance

3/4 teaspoon salt

DIRECTIONS

1. Season chicken with salt.
2. Layer fennel in the bottom of the slow cooker. Drizzle with vinegar. Then add chicken. Drizzle with oil. Top with carrots, herbs and orange slices.
3. Cook on low for 6-8 hours.
4. Shred meat and serve.

SLOW COOKER
THAI PEANUT CHICKEN

INGREDIENTS

- 1 1/2 pounds chicken breast
- 1 cup full fat coconut milk
- 1/3 cup smooth peanut butter
- 2 tablespoons honey
- 1 tablespoon rice vinegar
- 1 tablespoon grated fresh ginger
- 1 tablespoon lime juice
- 1/2 teaspoon salt

PREP TIME 10 MINUTES

COOK TIME 8 HOURS

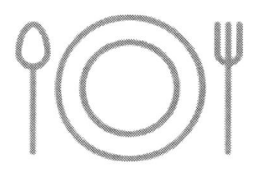

SERVES 6

DIRECTIONS

1. Season chicken with salt
2. In a small bowl, combine the rest of the seasoning ingredients.
3. Place chicken in slow cooker and pour the mixture over chicken.
4. Cook on low for 6-8 hours.
5. Shred meat and serve.

SLOW COOKER BOURBON CHICKEN

INGREDENTS

3 pounds chicken thighs

1/3 cup fresh apple juice

1/4 cup soy sauce or coconut amino

1/4 cup Bourbon

1/4 cup water

3 tablespoons apple cider vinegar

3 tablespoons honey

1 teaspoon grated fresh ginger

1/2 teaspoon salt

PREP TIME
10 MINUTES

COOK TIME
8 HOURS

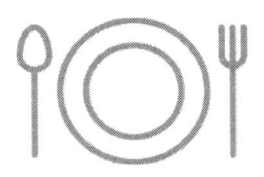

SERVES
8

DIRECTIONS

1. Season chicken with salt
2. In a small bowl, combine the rest of the seasoning ingredients.
3. Place chicken in slow cooker and pour the mixture over chicken.
4. Cook on low for 6-8 hours.
5. Shred meat and serve.

SLOW COOKER CHICKEN TIKKA MASALA

INGREDENTS

1 1/2 pounds chicken breast

1 15-ounce can full fat coconut milk

1 cup chicken broth

1/2 cup chopped fresh cilantro

2 teaspoons grated fresh turmeric of 1 teaspoon dried

2 teaspoons garam masala

1 teaspoon dried coriander

1 teaspoon cumin

1/2 teaspoon salt

PREP TIME
10 MINUTES

COOK TIME
8 HOURS

SERVES
6

DIRECTIONS

1. In a small bowl, combine all seasoning ingredients.

2. Place chicken in slow cooker and pour the mixture over chicken.

3. Cook on low for 6-8 hours.

4. Shred meat and serve.

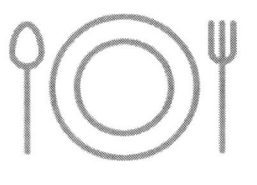

SLOW COOKER
HAWAIIAN PINEAPPLE CHICKEN

PREP TIME
10 MINUTES

COOK TIME
8 HOURS

SERVES
6

INGREDIENTS

1 1/2 pounds chicken breast

2 cups fresh pineapple chunks

3 tablespoons honey

2 tablespoons soy sauce

1/4 cup maple syrup

1 tablespoon grated fresh ginger

DIRECTIONS

1. In a small bowl, combine all seasoning ingredients.
2. Place chicken and pineapple chunks in slow cooker and pour the mixture over.
3. Cook on low for 6-8 hours.
4. Shred meat and serve.

SLOW COOKER MONGOLIAN BEEF

INGREDIENTS

2 pounds grass-fed beef stew meat

2 large carrots, peeled and sliced

1/2 cup water

1/2 cup soy sauce or coconut amino

1/3 cup beef broth

3 tablespoons honey

2 tablespoons butter

2 teaspoons grated fresh ginger

PREP TIME
15 MINUTES

COOK TIME
7 HOURS

SERVES
6

DIRECTIONS

1. In a pan, brown the beef in batches with butter.

2. Add browned beef and the rest of the ingredients to the slow cooker. Mix well.

3. Cover and cook on low for 6 hours. Add carrots and cook for another 1 hour.

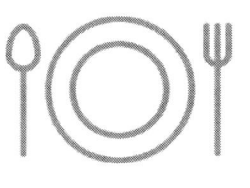

SLOW COOKER BEEF BOURGUIGNON

PREP TIME
15 MINUTES

COOK TIME
8 HOURS

SERVES
6

INGREDIENTS

- 2 pounds grass-fed beef stew meat, cut into bite-size
- 2 large carrots, peeled and sliced
- 1 small rutabaga, peeled and diced
- 2 cups bone broth
- 2 sprigs of fresh rosemary
- 2 bay leaves
- 2 tablespoons butter
- 2 tablespoons Dijon Mustard
- 1 teaspoon salt

DIRECTIONS

1. Season the beef with salt.
2. In a pan, brown the beef in batches with butter.
3. Add browned beef and the rest of the ingredients to the slow cooker. Mix well.
4. Cover and cook on low for 8 hours

SLOW COOKER
CLASSIC POT ROAST

INGREDENTS

4 pounds boneless chuck roast

1 cup beef broth

4 large carrots, peeled and sliced

2 celery stick cut into pieces (omit if can't tolerate)

2 onions, quartered (omit if can't tolerate)

1 sprig thyme

2 bay leaves

1 1/2 teaspoon salt

PREP TIME
15 MINUTES

COOK TIME
8 HOURS

SERVES
12

DIRECTIONS

1. Season the beef with salt.

2. In a pan, brown the beef on both sides.

3. Place the vegetables in the slow cooker, followed by the beef, herbs and broth.

4. Cover and cook on low for 8 hours.

5. Shred meat and serve with liquid in the slow cooker.

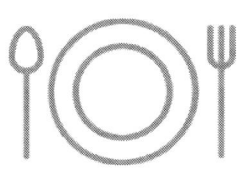

SLOW COOKER
ITALIAN ROASTED BEEF

PREP TIME
15 MINUTES

COOK TIME
8 HOURS

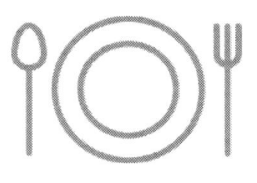

SERVES
6

INGREDIENTS

2 pounds beef round roast

1 small onion, sliced (omit if can't tolerate)

1/2 cup beef broth

1/2 cup red wine

1 teaspoon dried basil

1 teaspoon salt

1/2 teaspoon dried thyme

DIRECTIONS

1. Season the beef with salt.
2. In a pan, brown the beef on both sides.
3. Add beef broth and red wine to the slow cooker. Add the beef and sprinkle the spices on top. Top with onion slices.
4. Cover and cook on low for 8 hours.
5. Shred meat and serve with liquid in the slow cooker.

SLOW COOKER
MINTY LAMB SHANKS

INGREDENTS

2 large lamb shanks

2 tablespoons butter

1 teaspoon salt

For the sauce:

1 large bunch fresh mint, leaves only

1 teaspoon apple cider vinegar

1/2 teaspoon honey

PREP TIME
10 MINUTES

COOK TIME
5 HOURS

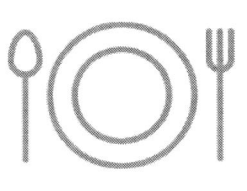

DIRECTIONS

1. Season the lamb with salt.

2. In a pan, brown the lamb.

3. Add lamb to slow cooker. Cover and cook on high for 5 hours. Shred the meat.

4. Use a blender or food processor to combine the sauce ingredients and serve over meat.

SERVES
4

SLOW COOKER LAMB CURRY

PREP TIME
10 MINUTES

COOK TIME
8 HOURS

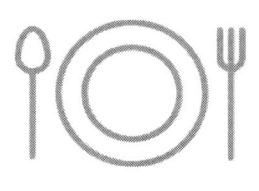

SERVES
6

INGREDIENTS

2 pounds bone-in lamb shoulder, sliced along the bones

1 15-ounce coconut milk

1/8 cup rice vinegar

2 slices fresh ginger

2 tablespoons butter

1 teaspoon salt

1 teaspoon curry powder (or replace with 1/2 teaspoon turmeric if can't tolerate)

1/2 teaspoon ground coriander

1/2 teaspoon ground cumin

1/8 teaspoon ground cloves

1/8 teaspoon cinnamon

DIRECTIONS

1. Season the lamb with salt.
2. In a pan, brown the lamb in batches with butter.
3. Add browned lamb and the rest of the ingredients to the slow cooker. Mix well.
4. Cover and cook on low for 8 hours.
5. Shred meat and serve with liquid in the slow cooker.

SLOW COOKER
APPLE SQUASH LAMB STEW

INGREDENTS

2 pounds lamb stew meat, cut into bite-size

1/2 medium butternut squash, peeled and diced

2 large apples, peeled, cored and cut into wedges

3 cups beef broth

2 tablespoons butter

2 tablespoons chopped fresh sage leaves

2 teaspoon ground ginger

1 teaspoon salt

PREP TIME
10 MINUTES

COOK TIME
8 HOURS

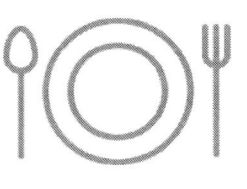

SERVES
6

DIRECTIONS

1. Season the lamb with salt.
2. In a pan, brown the lamb in batches with butter.
3. Add browned lamb and the rest of the ingredients to the slow cooker. Mix well.
4. Cover and cook on low for 8 hours.

SLOW COOKER
LEMON ROSEMARY LAMB

PREP TIME
10 MINUTES

COOK TIME
10 HOURS

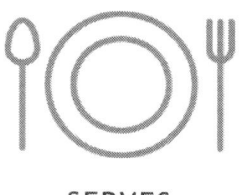

SERVES
8

INGREDIENTS

1 whole lamb leg, about 3-4 pounds

2 tablespoons olive oil

1 bunch of fresh rosemary leaves

Zest of 1 lemon

Juice of 1 lemon

DIRECTIONS

1. Make incisions on the leg and stuff rosemary in it. Rub the leg with olive oil and place the leg in the slow cooker.

2. Drizzle with lemon juice and top with lemon zest.

3. Cover and cook on low for 10 hours. Shred meat and serve.

SLOW COOKER
HONEY GINGER LIME PORK

INGREDENTS

2 pounds pork tenderloin

1 lime, juice only

1/2 cup honey

1/4 cup soy sauce or coconut amino

1 tablespoon Worcestershire sauce

1/2 teaspoon ground ginger

1/2 teaspoon salt

PREP TIME
10 MINUTES

COOK TIME
8 HOURS

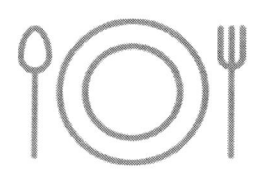

SERVES
6

DIRECTIONS

1. Rub the pork with salt and place in the slow cooker.
2. In a small bowl, combine the rest of the ingredients and pour over the pork.
3. Cover and cook on low for 6-8 hours.
4. Shred meat and serve.

SLOW COOKER
MAPLE BALSAMIC PORK

INGREDENTS

2 pounds pork tenderloin

1 cup water

1/2 cup balsamic vinegar

1/3 cup maple syrup

2 tablespoons soy sauce or coconut amino

1/2 teaspoon salt

PREP TIME
10 MINUTES

COOK TIME
8 HOURS

SERVES
6

DIRECTIONS

1. Rub the pork with salt and place in the slow cooker.
2. In a small bowl, combine the rest of the ingredients and pour over the pork.
3. Cover and cook on low for 6-8 hours.
4. Shred meat and serve.

SLOW COOKER
APPLE ROSEMARY PORK ROAST

INGREDIENTS

1 whole pork shoulder roast, about 3 pounds

3 medium apples, peeled, cored and chopped

1 cup chicken broth

6 sprigs rosemary

4 sprigs basil, leaves only

1 tablespoons chopped chives

1/2 teaspoon salt

PREP TIME
10 MINUTES

COOK TIME
10 HOURS

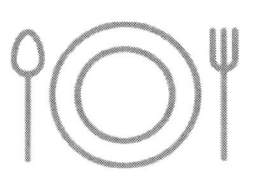

SERVES
9

DIRECTIONS

1. Rub the pork shoulder with salt and place in the slow cooker.
2. Add herbs and top with apples.
3. Cover and cook on low for 8-10 hours.
4. Shred meat and serve.

SLOW COOKER CUBAN PORK

PREP TIME 10 MINUTES

COOK TIME 10 HOURS

SERVES 9

INGREDIENTS

- 1 whole pork shoulder roast, about 3 pounds
- 1 small onion, sliced (omit if can't tolerate)
- 1/2 cup fresh orange juice
- 1/2 cup fresh lime juice
- 2 tablespoons extra virgin olive oil
- 1 teaspoon salt
- 1 teaspoon cumin
- 1 teaspoon dried oregano

DIRECTIONS

1. Rub the pork shoulder with salt and place in the slow cooker. Top with onion.
2. In a small bowl, combine the rest of the ingredients. and pour over the pork.
3. Cover and cook on low for 8-10 hours.
4. Shred meat and serve.

Printed in Great Britain
by Amazon